ALLE ZEIT WACH · 1842

Interaction Between Mental and Physical Illness

Needed Areas of Research

Edited by R. Öhman H. L. Freeman
A. Franck Holmkvist S. Nielzén

In Collaboration with Members
of the EMRC Study Group on Mental Illness Research
E. E. Anttinen, R. J. Daly, T. Helgason, H. Hippius,
R. Sadoun and E. A. Sand

With a Foreword by H. Danielsson

Springer-Verlag
Berlin Heidelberg New York
London Paris Tokyo

Professor ROLF ÖHMAN
University Hospital
Department of Psychiatry
S-221 85 Lund

Dr. ANNIKA FRANCK HOLMKVIST
University Hospital
Department of Psychiatry
S-221 85 Lund

Professor HUGH L. FREEMAN
The British Journal of Psychiatry
17 Belgrave Square
GB-London SWIX 8PG

Dr. SÖREN NIELZÉN
University Hospital
Department of Psychiatry
S-221 85 Lund

With 23 Figures and 12 Tables

ISBN-13:978-3-642-73995-8 e-ISBN-13:978-3-642-73993-4
DOI: 10.1007/978-3-642-73993-4

Softcover reprint of the hardcover 1st edition 1989

2125/3130-543210 – Printed on acid-free paper

European Science Foundation

This volume arises from the work of the Study Group on Mental Illness, a priority activity of the European Medical Research Councils (EMRC), which in turn is one of the five Standing Committees of the European Science Foundation (ESF). The EMRC, like the other ESF Committees, which cover the natural sciences, space science, humanities, and the social sciences, brings together the research councils and academies of 18 European countries. Under the auspices of EMRC and ESF generally, European scientists work on topics of common concern, co-ordinate the use of expensive facilities, and discover and define new endeavours that would benefit from a co-operative approach. Other typical work in the field studied in this book includes the European Training Programme in Brain and Behaviour Research, run by the ESF, closely linked with EMRC. In 1987 it brought together 500 young scientists from all over Europe in its Fellowships and residential courses.

Further information on EMRC and ESF activities can be obtained from:

European Science Foundation
1 Quai Lezay Marnésia
6700 Strasbourg, France

Foreword

The group of European Medical Research Councils (EMRC) was formed in 1971 and became a Standing Committee of the European Science Foundation (ESF) in 1975. EMRC is an association of medical research councils or equivalent organizations in Western Europe. The National Institutes of Health, the Israel Academy of Sciences, and the European Office of WHO are associated with EMRC and take an active part in its activities. The main aims of EMRC are to exchange information on the research policies pursued by its member organizations and to initiate and stimulate international cooperation in biomedical research. Since this research is highly international in itself, EMRC concentrates its activities on furthering international collaboration in those fields where it can play a significant role as a complement of existing channels. Mental illness research has been judged by EMRC to fulfill these criteria.

After a survey of the activities of the member organizations in mental illness research, EMRC decided in 1978 to set up a study group to analyze areas where EMRC could contribute. As a result of the work of the study group, five workshops have been arranged to define present knowledge in some specific areas and to delineate research needs. The present volume contains the proceedings of the fifth workshop, held in 1987 and dealing with interactions between mental and physical illness. EMRC hopes that this volume will contribute both to intensified research and to research cooperation on mental illnesses.

HENRY DANIELSSON
Chairman of EMRC

Preface

The dichotomy between mental and physical illness has deep roots in the traditions of academic medicine and in the public view of health problems in general. The progressive delineation of psychiatry from somatic medicine, notably neurology and internal medicine, has in many ways prevented integration of knowledge, as much from a clinical as from a scientific perspective. The conceptualization of body-mind interaction has not been truly updated.

Undoubtedly, the development of psychiatry has added diagnostic and therapeutic qualities with significant impact on our strategies for ameliorating severe psychiatric illness. During the same period, however, the area between psychiatry and other medical disciplines has suffered from lack of interest, priorities, and resources, or even from neglect. Clinical signs, symptoms, and syndromes which clearly signal interaction between somatic dysfunction and the mental process have too often been left aside, untouched by necessary interdisciplinary discussion, education, critical review, and research.

Psychosomatic states in the form of somatization of anxiety, aggression and sexuality, chronic pain syndromes, sleep disorders, and gastrointestinal, dermatological, or gynaecological problems, illustrate areas where medical professional interest has been insufficient or absent. Many of these problems have been left to paramedical or even lay intervention. The present wave of "alternative medicine" (psychologically or somatically orientated) may in fact be to a large extent a logical consequence of neglect by both the medical profession and the public health system. The public need for understanding and acceptance of body-mind interaction has not been adequately evaluated.

During recent years, in a series of conferences and publications, the European Medical Research Council (EMRC) has tried to identify needed areas of research and professional support. With the background outlined above, it was logical that the topic selected for the EMRC symposium in 1987 held in Lund, Sweden, was "Interaction between Mental and Physical Illness." The EMRC has directed the work through a program committee headed by Tómas Helgason, and it has been a pleasure for the local organizers and editors of this volume to fulfil its intentions.

The EMRC symposium was structured in the form of both contributions by invited speakers and discussants and by general discussion among the participants. For purposes of clarity, the editors have incorporated these contributions and opinions into the reviews and summarized discussion. This volume should therefore be seen as a contribution by all participants of the symposium.

The organizers and editors also extend their gratitude to all those who made this symposium successful. Monica Pardon has skilfully administered the arrangements, editing, and, correspondence. Tómas Helgason and the officers of the EMRC undertook the contacts with the national research organizations during the preparation of the meeting. Through Henry Danielsson, the Swedish Medical Research Council provided essential encouragement and financial support. AB LEO/Pharmacia and AB Essex are also gratefully acknowledged for promoting the symposium with logistical support and grants.

The Editors

Contents

List of Contributors

You will find the address of each first mentioned author at the beginning of the respective contribution

Psychiatric Consequences of Physical Illness – Clinical Aspects

J.-O. OTTOSSON

In principle, physical illness can lead to mental consequences in two ways – either via cerebral lesions or via the experience of being physically ill and the patient's psychological reaction to that. We may therefore speak of both somatogenic and psychogenic mental consequences of physical illness.

Somatogenic Mental Consequences

A cerebral lesion is here defined as the pathological function of neurons: lesions may be biochemical and reversible or structural and irreversible. In respect of their origin, they may be divided into histogenic, i.e., caused by pathological processes in the central nervous system (CNS), or chemogenic, i.e., caused by alteration of the blood flow through the CNS (Fig. 1).

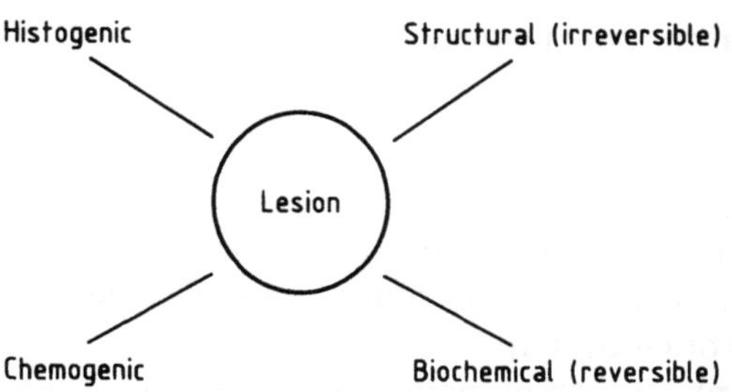

Fig. 1. A cerebral lesion

Forms of Exogenous Reaction

That there was a characteristic mental picture for every physical disease was a belief that was long held, for instance by Kraepelin. It was not until 1912 that Bonhoeffer (1912) described the various forms of exogenous reaction (*exogene Reaktionstypen*) and emphasized their lack of specificity, universality, and independence of the nature of the underlying physical disease. He differentiated acute and chronic forms of the psycho-organic syndrome. The acute syndrome

Department of Psychiatry, Sahlgren Hospital, University of Gothenburg,
S-41345 Gothenburg

Interaction Between Mental and Physical Illness
Edited by R. Öhman et al.

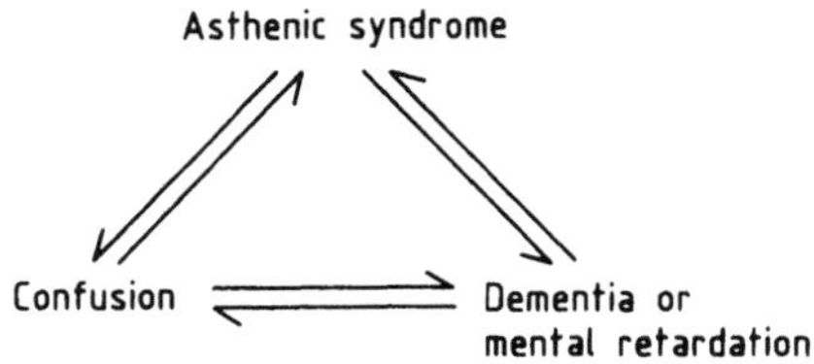

Fig. 2. The asthenic syndrome

consists of confusion and arises when a somatogenic factor rapidly produces a diffuse lesion. The chronic syndrome emerges when diffuse lesions are produced slowly and insidiously, and consists of dementia – intellectual and personality deterioration – or mental retardation dependent upon when the lesion occurs in relation to the individual's phase of development. These psycho-organic syndromes are now recognized as typical manifestations of diffuse cerebral lesions, but a third form is even more common. Bonhoeffer described *emotionell-hyperästhetische Schwächezustände*, which is described today as the asthenic or asthenic-depressive syndrome; it consists of the following symptoms:

- Fatiguability
- Affective lability
- Irritability
- Depression-dysphoria
- Disturbance of attention, concentration, and memory
- Sensitivity to sound and light
- Symptoms of tensions
- Insomnia

The asthenic syndrome may be the only sign of a diffuse cerebral lesion but, may also be a transitional syndrome to and from the other forms of exogenous reaction (Fig. 2). These conditions often overlap.

However, the pendulum towards describing nonspecific forms of exogenous reaction may have swung too far, since a finer discrimination is sometimes possible and may give clues to the underlying physical illness. For instance, there is a fairly good correlation between the localization of the pathological process in the CNS and the psychopathological syndrome. This is close enough to justify the syndromes deriving their names in some cases from the area of the brain that is referred to. The following are focal lesional syndromes:

- Frontal lobe syndrome
- Temporal lobe syndrome
- Parietal lobe syndrome
- Parkinson's disease
- Huntington's disease
- Tourette's syndrome
- Wernicke-Korsakoff's syndrome

Recent investigations have demonstrated two principal patterns of neuropsychological deterioration within the dementias (Cummings 1986). A cortical pattern is characterized by intellectual decline including deterioration of language, learning, perception, calculation, and praxis, and is manifested by aphasia, a cortical type of amnesia, agnosia, acalculia, and apraxia. A subcortical pattern includes disturbances of motivation, mood, attention, and arousal, as evidenced by psychomotor slowing, an axial type of amnesia, affective and emotional disorders, and difficulties with strategy-formation and problem-solving. Anatomically, the cortical pattern is produced by diseases mainly involving the association cortex of the cerebral hemispheres and the medial temporal lobes, whereas the subcortical pattern occurs in disorders of the basal ganglia, thalamus, brain stem, and also the frontal cortex, which has dense connections with the caudate nucleus. The striatum also receives projections from limbic structures, indicating that the cortical-subcortical division is not an absolute one. Neurochemically, acetylcholine plays an essential role in cortical neurotransmission, whereas a variety of neurotransmitters including dopamine, serotonin, noradrenalin, GABA, and acetylcholine are utilized in subcortical nuclei. Alzheimer's and Pick's disease are examples of cortical dementias, while the dementia syndromes associated with Huntington's and Parkinson's disease as well as with subcortical infarctions and infectious, metabolic, and neoplastic conditions exemplify subcortical dementias.

All these examples refer to histogenic lesions which at least in their early stages, may be more circumscribed than chemogenic lesions, which having arisen via the cerebral blood flow, are inevitably diffuse. However, even in such cases, the lesions may be more or less focal since brain areas vary in their sensitivity to chemogenic influences. For instance, the limbic forebrain or Papez circuit has a higher metabolic rate than the rest of the CNS, and is more sensitive to hypoxia. Cerebral lesions in survivors after suicide attempts by drowning, hanging, strangulation, or CO poisoning may therefore display typical axial amnesia as part of the Korsakoff syndrome. The sensitivity to thiamine deficiency also varies, being highest in the brain stem nuclei of the oculomuscular nerves, which explains some of the symptoms of Wernicke's encephalopathy (nystagmus and ophthalmoplegia). There may be more such correlations between lesion and psychopathology, which have not yet been described, and this is understandable, since they are masked by the nonspecific psycho-organic syndromes.

Classification Issues

In view of the fact that the asthenic is the most common of all psychopathological syndromes, it is remarkable that it has no heading of its own in the two most important classification systems in current use. In ICD-9 (WHO 1976) some of these cases may be classified as postconcussional syndrome (300C) and others as specified (310W) or unspecified nonpsychotic mental disturbance after cerebral lesion (310X). Neurasthenia (300F) is placed under neuroses and cannot be used when the cause is somatic.

Neither has the asthenic syndrome a heading of its own in DSM-III-R (American Psychiatric Association 1987). It belongs to a residual category (atypical or mixed organic brain syndrome 294.80) that does not meet the criteria for any other organic brain syndrome (delirium 293.00, dementia 294.10, amnestic syndrome 294.00, organic delusional syndrome 393.81, organic hallucinosis 293.82, organic affective syndrome 293.83, or organic personality syndrome 310.10). In the index of DSM-III-R, neurasthenia appears under dysthymic disorder which, however, cannot be used when the cause is somatic. It seems obvious that there are good reasons to revise the classification systems in order to give the asthenic syndrome the position it deserves. It should be used as a descriptive diagnosis and not as a nosological unity, but having established the descriptive diagnosis, an etiological dimension should be added. The asthenic syndrome may both be somatogenic and psychogenic; often, factors belonging to both categories contribute. As may be seen from the following, a list of the somatogenic factors underlying the asthenic syndrome covers most of internal medicine:

- Post-infectious
- Post-concussional
- Hypoxia
- Nutritional deficiency
  - B_{12}
  - Folic acid
  - Thiamine
  - Hypoglycemia
- Endocrinopathies
- Malignancies
  - Carcinoma pancreatis
- Electrolyte disturbances
- Toxins
  - Endotoxins
  - Exotoxins
  - Alcohol
  - Drugs
  - CO
  - Heavy metals
  - Hydrocarbons
- Neuronal degeneration
- Intracranial expansive processes
- Cardiovascular disease
- Systemic diseases

Psychogenic Consequences of Physical Illness

All diseases, if they are not of a trivial nature, give rise to a psychogenic response which usually takes the form of a crisis reaction; the course of this reaction depends on the nature of the physical illness, but also on whether or not mechanisms of defence are elicited. As a result of denial, the experience of anxiety may be reduced and a state of anosognosia may develop in which the patient does not take the necessary measures to obtain medical help. A close correlation has been demonstrated between the activation of mechanisms of defence and a patient's delay in seeking treatment for mammary cancer (Gyllensköld 1973).

The psychological reaction may also have repercussions on the physical illness. For instance, in both infectious diseases and malignancies this may be exerted by immunological mechanisms and in ischemic heart disease (IHD) by influence on clotting time, platelet aggregation, cathecholamine output, level of blood lipids, and blood pressure.

Misinterpreted Mental Symptoms

Mental symptoms are sometimes erroneously attributed to somatoform disorders according to DSM-III-R. The Briquet or polysymptomatic form of hysteria is usually regarded as a mental disorder, but a recent study (Orenstein et al. 1986) showed a relationship between the Briquet syndrome and polycystic ovary disease. This is a state with an elevated plasma level of luteinizing and low level of follicle-stimulating hormone, as well as an elevated prolactin level sometimes. This pattern may be consistent with a hypothalamic dopaminergic deficiency. This finding suggests that Briquet's syndrome may include subtle physiological and anatomical abnormalities and that categorical distinctions between physical and psychological disorders may be arbitrary.

Mental symptoms can also be erroneously attributed to physical illness. Three examples, all connected with Sweden, may illustrate this probably common strategy of finding a medical solution to difficult life situations. According to the Story of San Michele, in Paris about 100 years ago, Dr. Axel Munthe established the diagnosis of colitis in his aristocratic female patients, giving them an acceptable explanation of their nervous symptoms and himself an income with which he could later buy San Michele. About 50 years ago, at the time of World War II when cars were fueled by wood-gas, many people with a variety of psychiatric disorders were diagnosed as suffering from chronic CO intoxication. Yet, in very few, if any, was the diagnosis correct, though they got their invalid pension and the symptoms subsequently diminished. We now have a new Swedish disease – oral galvanism or micromercurialism – in which people consider themselves intoxicated with mercury from the amalgam fillings, while up to now, no convincing evidence has been presented to support such a statement. Diagnoses change, but the need to adopt a sick role seems to be constant.

Needed Areas of Research

Neurobiology

Specific psychopathological patterns which are now masked by the nonspecific asthenic syndrome, confusion, dementia or mental retardation should be unmasked by careful mapping of the symptoms and course of individual cases. Possibilities would then open up to study the neurobiological basis of various psychopathological syndromes while early diagnosis would be facilitated, preferably before the biochemical lesion has developed into a structural lesion.

Clarification of the putative association between various symptoms and amalgam fillings also needs to be investigated.

Psychogenic Factors

Many questions pertaining to the importance of the patient's mental state for the course of physical illness still need to be elucidated. Psychological factors in the care of the patient should also be studied with regard to their importance for the treatment of diseases. More specifically the following issues should be examined in future research.

- How does the mental state influence the course of infectious diseases, malignancies, and IHD?
- Through which psychoneuroimmunological, physiological, and biochemical mechanisms are these influences exerted?
- Is it important if defence mechanisms are elicited, i.e., whether or not the patient experiences anxiety?
- How can concurrent psychological treatment promote the effect of measures taken against the disease process?

There are many hypotheses in this area which need to be tested and preliminary results which need to be replicated. If verified, the case for considering psychological factors in the care of patients will not only be a matter of quality and humaneness, but also necessary prerequisite for an optimal outcome of medical treatment.

References

American Psychiatric Association (1987) Diagnostic and statistical manual of mental disorders, 3rd edn. APA, Washington DC

Bonhoeffer K (1912) Die Psychosen im befolge von akuten Infektionen, Allgemeinerkrankungen und inneren Erkrankungen. In: Aschaffenburg G (ed) Handbuch der Psychiatrie. Deuticke, Leipzig

Cummings JL (1986) Subcortical dementia. Neuropsychology, neuropsychiatry and pathophysiology. Br J Psychiatry 149:682–697

Gyllensköld K (1973) Cancerpatienters upplevelse av och anpassning till sin sjukdom. Thesis, Stockholm University

Orenstein H, Raskind MA, Wyllie D, Raskind WH, Soules MR (1986) Polysymptomatic complaints and Briquet's syndrome in polycystic ovary disease. Am J Psychiatry 143:768–771

WHO (1976) International classification of diseases, 9th revision. WHO, Geneva

Discussion of Professor Ottosson's Paper

D. GOLDBERG

While it is true that the category of "neurasthenia" has not been recognized by either ICD-10 or DSM-IIIR, I am not sure that this is important. The classifications of anxiety-related and mood disorders which are offered by either of these systems *do* allow us to classify the commonest sorts of patients seen in general medical settings – who are certainly patients with various combinations of symptoms of anxiety and depression.

There have been changes in both major systems of classification: in the DSM-IIIR system, one cannot now have a "generalized anxiety disorder" until one has been anxious for 6 months; while in ICD-10, states of "mixed anxiety depression" are classified as anxiety disorders unless the depressive symptoms reach a certain pitch of severity – when the patient is thought of as having an affective disorder. I have preferred to use a system of double diagnosis – so that a patient who satisfies criteria both for an anxiety state and a depressive illness is classified as having both illnesses. I am not as unhappy as Ottosson about using conventional diagnoses such as "major depressive episode" or "anxiety state" for the disorders seen on medical wards, since in my experience they are phenomenologically similar to such illnesses seen in community settings, and therefore attract the same descriptive labels.

I do not agree that the neurasthenic syndrome is distinctive and requires a separate category. Although the symptoms of fatigue, lack ef energy, and instability make up a cluster of related symptoms of equal severity, I regard them as representing a minor degree of anxiety/depression (Goldberg et al. 1987; Grayson et al. 1987). In China, where psychiatrists still use the concept of "neurasthenia", Kleinman and Kleinman (1985) showed that 93% of those receiving this label satisfied DSM-III criteria for depressive illness, and 69% satisfied the criteria for anxiety disorders. I do not think any useful purpose would be served by re-introducing the concept of neurasthenia.

The existence of many cases of psychiatric illness which are undetected by doctors working in general medical settings (for review, see Goldberg 1984) has resulted in us introducing two-stage screening strategies, in which the GHQ-28 and the CAGE questionnaire for alcoholism are used as screening tests; we then interview those with high scores, to form our own diagnostic

University of Manchester Department of Psychiatry, Withington Hospital, Manchester M2O 8LR, UK

Interaction Between Mental and Physical Illness
Edited by R. Öhman et al.

Table 1. Classification of relationships which exist between psychiatric and physical illness

	Diagnostic criteria
1. Physical illness with secondary psychiatric illness	1. All somatic symptoms can be attributed to physical illness 2. Treatment of the psychiatric illness will not remove the physical symptoms 3. The psychiatric illness would not have occurred without the physical illness
2. Physical illness with unrelated psychiatric illness	No aetiological link exists between the two: treatment of one would not affect the other
3. Somatized psychiatric illness	1. Consultation is for physical symptoms 2. Patient attributes all problems to a physical illness, or thinks symptoms constitute the problem 3. A psychiatric illness (DSM-III) is present 4. Treatment of the psychiatric illness would alleviate or remove the physical symptom (*all four must be satisfied*)
4. Entirely psychiatric illness	Either no somatic symptoms are present, or patient considers somatic symptoms are part of psychiatric illness

judgements about the nature of the illnesses seen. Furthermore, we have used a classification which tries to take account of the complex relationships which exist between psychiatric and physical illness. We recognize four relationships, as shown in Table 1.

The definition of "somatized psychiatric illness" includes two groups of patients: those who have coexisting physical disease (but the presenting symptoms are exacerbated by the psychiatric disorder), and those without demonstrable physical illness. We are aware that some authors have used the term to refer only to the latter group: but in the data to be presented here the term has been used as defined in Table 1.

It is of interest to see how this classification works in two quite different general medical settings: general practice and for patients admitted with severe physical illnesses to medical wards. These data are shown in Table 2.

It can be seen that physical illnesses with secondary psychiatric disorders are much more common in our medical wards, because the physical illnesses are often severe and life-threatening. However, "somatization" accounts for 57% of all psychiatric illnesses seen in primary care settings, and for 42.5% of those seen on the medical wards.

Bridges and Goldberg (1985, 1988) have shown that somatization is the most important reason why general practitioners tend to miss psychiatric illnesses – only 47.5% were detected by the family doctors. If the somatizers are divided by whether or not they have physical illness – then the family doctors detect 84% of those without, but only 33% of those with physical illness.

Table 2. Distribution of classification of relationships between psychiatric and physical illness, a comparison of patients on medical wards and primary care patients

	Medical ward patients		Primary care patients	
	All %	Psychiatric %	All %	Psychiatric %
Not psychiatrically ill (no disorder reaches DSM-III criteria)	80	–	67	–
Physical illness with secondary psychiatric illness	10	51	1	3.2
Unrelated physical and psychiatric illness	1.4	6.5	8	24
Somatisation	8.5	42.5	20	57
Entirely psychiatric illness	0	0	5	15
Total %	100	100	100	100
Total *n*	236	47	590	195

Table 3. Diagnostic breakdown of patients with high scores on the General Health Questionnaire 28 and supported by results of semistructured interview (from among consecutive patients admitted to the medical wards)

	%	*n*
Depression	39	42 }
Depression + anxiety state	25	27 } 81%
Anxiety state	17	18 }
Alcoholism	9	10
Heroin abuse	1	1
Somatization without physical disorder	4	4
Dementia	2	2
Other	3	3
		107

On the medical wards, approximately half the illnesses are not detected by the medical staff, and there is no tendency for the undetected illnesses to be milder than the detected illnesses in either setting. In the medical wards almost all the patients have a physical disease which seems to distract the physician from the psychiatric illness. We have shown that pure depressive illnesses are more likely to be detected than cases of both depression *and* anxiety state, even though the latter patients have more symptoms. We suspect that the way that medical students are taught about neurotic illness is responsible for the diagnostic stereotypes that are clearly in the minds of our medical colleagues.

We have therefore conducted a study in which medical students administrated the GHQ-28 to consecutive admissions to the medical wards, and carried out brief semistructured interviews with patients who had high scores (McGrath et al. 1986). These patients were later interviewed by the psychiatrists, who made their own diagnoses of the patients.

Results from two recent studies carried out in our Department have been combined to give the diagnostic breakdown shown in Table 3.

Much as I admire the classification offered by Bonhoeffer that Ottosson has recommended, I do not find it of use in practice, and prefer to retain the concepts shown in Table 3. It should be emphasized that patients with acute brain syndromes did occur, but could not be included in this study since they were not well enough to cooperate with the screening procedure.

Recommendations for Further Research

There should be further evaluation of the effects of offering psychiatric treatment for the psychiatric illnesses seen in general medical settings. Outcome measures should include economic measures: "medical offset" refers to the costs of medical investigations which may not need to be carried out if the patient receives more appropriate treatment.

In conjunction with WHO in Geneva, we have produced instructional videotapes for physicians on our detection and treatment of depression on medical wards.[1] These videotapes are available in both English and French. It is essential that other workers experiment with these tapes, to discover whether or not depressive illnesses could be detected and treated by the usual medical staff in their settings.

Somatization remains an important way in which psychiatric illness presents in general medical settings. It is important that we produce educational packages dealing with the management of somatized psychiatric illnesses for general practitioners and physicians. Furthermore, such packages should then be evaluated in clinical settings to discover the optimal management of these common and important disorders.

References

Bridges KW, Goldberg DP (1985) Somatic presentations of DSM-III psychiatric disorders in primary care. J Psychosom Res 29:563–569

Goldberg DP (1984) The recognition of psychiatric illness by non-psychiatrists. Aust NZ J Psychiatry 18:128–134

Goldberg DP, Bridges KW (1988) Somatic presentations of psychiatric illness in primary care settings. J Psychosom Res 32:137–144

[1] Available from Tavistock Publications, 11 New Fetter Lane, London EC4P 4EE, UK

Goldberg DP, Bridges KW, Duncan-Jones P, Grayson D (1987) Dimensions of neurosis seen in primary care settings. Psychol Med 17:461–470

Grayson D, Bridges K, Duncan-Jones P, Goldberg DP (1987) The relationship between symptoms and diagnoses of minor psychiatric disorder in general practice. Psychol Med 17:933–942

Kleinman A, Kleinman J (1985) The inter-connections in Chinese society aming culture, depressive experiences, and the meanings of pain. In: Kleinman A, Good B (eds) Culture and depression. University of California Press, Los Angeles

McGrath G, Godbert K, Goldberg DP, Stone K, Tantam D (1986) Use of a general medical setting to teach medical students about neurosis. Med Educ 20:222–227

Psychiatric Consequences of Physical Illness – Clinical Aspects: Discussion

H. HELMCHEN

The diagnostic concepts in ICD-9 associated with the topic psychiatric consequences of physical illness are summarized in Fig. 1. A narrow definition would restrict the topic to "organic" states, such as delirium. However, our understanding of the psychiatric consequences of physical illness would be increased by including clinical experiences and research results from a broader perspective of the soma-psyche relationship. This is represented in the middle and right-hand parts of the figure. Some reasons for such a view are that:

1. Physical illnesses are mainly treated in medical departments, which do not involve psychiatry. In that setting, their mental consequences will be seen only as epiphenomena or disturbing complications, and these are often treated without psychiatric intervention or insight.
2. The typical psychopathology of organic brain syndromes, i.e., delirium and dementia, has been broadened, since mild, incipient, or reversible brain disorders have been added to the more severe conditions.
3. The diagnostic study of both structural and functional brain disturbances is now being approached in more sophisticated ways – in qualitative, spatial, and temporal terms.

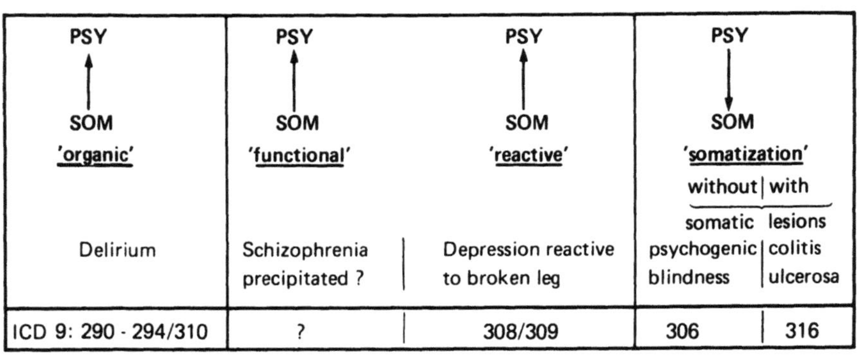

Fig. 1. Types of association between psychopathological and somatic conditions

Psychiatrische Klinik und Poliklinik, Freie Universität Berlin, Eschenallee 3, D-1000 Berlin 19 (West)

Interaction Between Mental and Physical Illness
Edited by R. Öhman et al.

The need for future research in this area is important for two sets of reasons.

First, because of higher average life expectancy, increasing exposure to possibly pathogenic environmental influences, and the hope of a therapeutic breakthrough for dementia during the next decade, it has become necessary to diagnose even incipient or mild dementia. In such cases, existing clinical-psychopathological diagnostic studies can often only yield a possible diagnostic decision with greater or lesser degrees of probability. It is especially important to differentiate such states from normal aging, as well as from depressive disorders, i.e., the problem of depressive pseudodementia. On the other hand, existing neuropsychological tests have strong limitations, with respect both to their time-consuming nature and their limited applicability. They are also insensitive towards mild disturbances, particularly those of affect and daily activities.

Thus, it is important to improve our diagnostic techniques, e.g., by including investigation of nonverbal behavior or of neuro- and psychophysiological disturbances. The development of broadly applicable neuropsychological tests for the quantification of organic brain syndromes will also be a prerequisite for the evaluation of therapy. Furthermore, the generally fairly global psychopathological diagnosis of dementia or organic brain syndrome should be made more precise by recording disturbances of single, neuropsychological components. This is necessary in order to differentiate these syndromes quantitatively by profiles of various disturbances of performance. Finally, greater cooperation is desirable between psychiatrists and physicians who may be responsible for the management of physical illnesses that are prone to mental consequences.

A second area of concern for why such neuropsychological diagnostic research is needed is represented by the psychopathological consequences of minimal cerebral dysfunction (MCD), particularly if that dysfunction is due to perinatal or early childhood brain lesions. Such lesions are estimated to occur in about 10% of the general population, but the frequency is perhaps at least twice as high in the population with "personality" and "neurotic disorders." If so, early brain lesions would be a major vulnerability factor underlying such disorders later in life. The diagnosis of specific neuropsychological deficits could have a great impact on the views taken by society of such conditions. More specifically, it would help in substituting or at least complementing psychodynamically orientated therapy with training in specific habilitative tasks and defined skills. In this field also, close and lasting cooperation should be expanded between obstetricians, neonatologists, neuropediatricians, child and adolescent psychiatrists, and adult psychiatrists. This is important not only to improve diagnosis, but also for the prospective investigation of the psychopathological consequences of such minimal brain lesions and the reactions to them in terms of compensation and coping. There have been very few convincing studies in this specific field, although many longitudinal and high-risk studies are reported in selected populations, for example, among the mentally retarded and children of parents with endogeneous psychoses.

Better neuropsychological, neurophysiological, and psychophysiological techniques for the diagnosis of mild, but perhaps very circumscribed psychopathological consequences of small brain lesions will probably make the borderline between the "organic" psychoses and other psychiatric diseases more permeable. This process should be heuristically productive. Thus, there is increasing evidence of such circumscribed deficits in schizophrenic patients. However, the significance of these deficits for the development of psychosis is as yet unknown, as is their relationship to definable brain lesions or dysfunctions (Helmchen and Henn 1987). In this connection, two important questions have to be answered:

- Are some of these deficits under genetic control? And if so, which ones?
- How does such a trait interact with environmental influences? And in that case, with which ones?

The same questions should also be put in connection with the "organic" psychoses. For example, there is evidence that not only the risk of becoming an alcoholic, but also the morbidity risk of different bodily organs, including the brain, from the influence of alcohol is genetically determined (Propping et al. 1981; Zerbin-Rüdin 1984). These considerations were also raised with regard to neurosyphilis in its time. Because of the curability of that disease, however, general paresis has lost its significance as a basic paradigm for psychiatric conceptualization. But this paradigm will probably be revitalized by the AIDS epidemic, because AIDS also affects the brain in the majority of infected people, has a long-lasting course, can be followed from the beginning in many patients, and unfortunately, is not likely to disappear in the foreseeable future. Public concern, the great need for care, and the development of cures for these patients provide an opportunity to test the old paradigm of general paresis on a new methodological level. This will be possible through interdisciplinary cooperation among infectious disease specialists, immunologists ("biological coping"), and neurobiologists, as well as through the application of measuring instruments for psychopathology and of brain imaging in prospective follow-up.

There are two further points with regard to these more technical aspects.

First, the development of brain imaging techniques, such as cranial computer tomography (CCT), nuclear magnetic resonance tomography (NMR-T), single photon emission computer tomography (SPECT), positron emission tomography (PET), and brain electrical activity mapping (BEAM) have made the invisible visible in vivo, particularly some of the more subtle structural and functional aspects of the living brain. There will be further rapid development from more global techniques, such as the 133 Xenon-SPECT for the measurement of regional cerebral blood flow (rCBF), to more specific measurements of localized brain metabolism, or even of spatial distribution of specific receptors and their activity by PET or NMR spectroscopy. Such results have already been reported for dopamine receptors in schizophrenics, and many others are to come (Sedvall et al. 1986).

With regard to the present topic, an in vivo replication of the finding that the serotonin concentration in defined brain regions is increased in comatose states of different origins, supports the hypothesis that such an increase could be at least one of the common pathogenetic pathways for the psychopathological consequences of acute brain syndromes (Jellinger et al. 1978; Jellinger and Riederer 1983). Bonhoeffer called this the "etiological connection" (*ätiologisches Zwischenglied*) between different somatic origins and fairly uniform psychopathological syndromes or "reaction types" (Bonhoeffer 1912).

Although these techniques yield results based on digital data, they are usually presented to the clinician as analog pictures, probably because clinicians are more accustomed to seeing and interpreting pictures than quantitative data. However, especially with respect to psychiatry, the necessary recognition of subtle morphological or functional lesions is often impossible from such analogous and even colored pictures. Therefore, there is a need to develop software for differentiated quantitative evaluation of such data and for systematically performed clinical investigations.

Second, although the application of these techniques is expensive, it can be justified for two reasons: its goal should be the definition of precise parameters of unequivocal brain lesions that correlate highly with, and thus validate practical and routinely applicable clinical tests. Better pathogenetic understanding as well as clinically more differentiated diagnosis of the psychiatric consequences of physical illness will improve prevention and therapy of these disorders and relieve the excessive burden on the patient, his family, and society.

References

Bonhoeffer K (1912) Die Psychosen im Gefolge von aktuellen Infektionen. In: Aschaffenburg G (ed) Handbuch der Psychiatrie, special part III/1. Deuticke, Leipzig, pp 1–118

Helmchen H, Henn F (eds) (1987) Biological perspectives of schizophrenia. Wiley, Chichester p 354

Jellinger K, Riederer P (1983) Zentrale Neurotransmitter bei zerebraler Ischämie und Hirninfarkt. Fortschr Neurol Psychiatr 51:91–123

Jellinger K, Riederer P, Rausch WD, Kothbauer P (1978) Brain monoamines in hepatic encephalopathy and other types of metabolic coma. J Neural Transm [Suppl] 14:103–120

Propping P, Krüger J, Mark N (1981) Genetic disposition to alcoholism. An EEG-study in alcoholics and their relatives. Hum Genet 59:51–59

Sedvall G, Farde L, Persson A, Wiesel FA (1986) Imaging of neurotransmitter receptors in the living human brain. Arch Gen Psychiatry 43:995–1005

Zerbin-Rüdin E (1984) Alkoholismus, Anlage und Umwelt. In: Zang KD (ed) Klinische Genetik des Alkoholismus. Kohlhammer, Stuttgart, pp 29–46

Epilepsy as a Model for Psychopathology

T. G. Bolwig

Although neurobiology plays an increasingly important role in psychiatry, we stand merely at the threshold of understanding at least part of the interface of behaviour and its neural substrates and largely ignore perhaps the most dramatic expression of that relationship. In the older textbooks, epilepsy, along with schizophrenia and affective illness, formed the triad of major psychiatric disorders referred to as "insanity." Since the introduction of EEG, though, epilepsy has been a disturbance belonging to the domain of neurologists, while psychiatrists have concentrated more on understanding the cerebral substrate of the major psychoses. In the case of epilepsy, with its obvious physical aspects, those of a psychiatric nature have been largely overlooked. Many neurologists have made major contributions to knowledge of the behavioural aspects of epilepsy, but they have not focused on the psychiatric features of their patients' conditions. On the other hand, for a long time, psychiatrists have favoured purely psychological theories and treatment approaches, while ignoring the brain and anything that could be labelled a "brain disease" (Blumer 1984). It is surprising that even modern, biologically oriented psychiatrists do not seem to consider epilepsy to be within their field of expertise and interest.

However, with the development of new techniques such as computerized EEG and methods for measuring regional cerebral blood flow (rCBF) and metabolism, a new view among psychiatrists of the neuropsychiatric aspects of epilepsy has inspired a number of research projects and papers. During the past 7 years, three books have appeared covering the psychiatric aspects of epilepsy (Reynolds and Trimble 1981; Blumer 1984; Trimble and Bolwig 1986).

Among the many reasons for studying epilepsy in relation to psychiatric disorders is the unique possibility of observing a connection between psychopathology and organic brain disturbances and thereby having a better chance than in any other condition to throw light on the pathophysiology of a neuropsychiatric disease. The bias against any relationship between epilepsy and psychiatric disturbances presupposes that psychiatric disorders are considered shameful and intractable. Yet nobody refrains from mentioning that there are malignant forms of hypertension, simply because that would give benign hypertension a bad name and blemish those who suffer from the disease (Blumer

Department of Psychiatry, Rigshospitalet, Blegdamsvej 9, DK-2100 Copenhagen

Interaction Between Mental and Physical Illness
Edited by R. Öhman et al.

1984). In fact, though concentrating on the malignant form of that illness, great progress has been made, and the number of those who suffer from the more critical forms have been drastically reduced.

The history of epilepsy is extremely interesting, and the description by Hippocrates in his book on "The Sacred Disease" naming epilepsy a hereditary illness seated in the brain is probably the first record of a battle between major beliefs by scientifically orientated physicians (Littré 1839–1861).

From antiquity, through the Middle Ages, the Renaissance, and up to the birth of modern neurology, epilepsy has either been considered the possession of spiritual or godly power, or has been connected with genius. Both the French school of neurology and central European psychiatrists at the turn of the century have discussed the phenomenon of hysteroepilepsy (Charcot 1877; Freud 1895; Janet 1907), and up to 1950 at least epilepsy was often discussed as being associated with personality disorders, for instance, in the influential textbook of psychiatry by Henderson and Gillespie (1950).

By definition, epilepsy is a chronic condition characterized by recurrent seizures. Patients who have seizures elicited by drugs such as neuroleptics and antidepressants or in connection with transient changes in cerebral function due to organic psychosyndromes, e.g., withdrawal phenomena, should not be classified as epileptic.

In their pioneering work Penfield and Jasper (1954) initiated a system of classification of seizures and epilepsy according to the (presumed) site of pathology in the brain. This provided a background of great importance for

Table 1. Classification of seizures (modified after Gastaut 1969)

Generalized seizures	Absence-Simple -Complex Myoclonic Infantile spasms Clonic seizures Tonic seizures Tonic-clonic seizures Atonic seizures Akinetic seizures	
Unilateral seizures		
Unclassified seizures		
Partial seizures	a) Simple or Elementary	– Motor Sensory Autonomic Compound
	b) Complex	– Impaired consciousness Cognitive symptoms Affective symptoms Psychosensory symptoms "Psychomotor" symptoms Compound
	c) Secondarily generalized	

those undertaking research into psychopathology, to whom a model became available for testing hypotheses concerning the relationship between brain and behaviour.

In 1969, Gastaut suggested a classification of various forms of seizures; a modification of this is given in Table 1.

Complex partial seizures (CPS) with a temporal EEG focus and with or without secondary generalization, are of interest to psychiatrists. In the complex form of these, changes in consciousness occur, and patients may present a variety of symptoms indicating impairment of mental functioning. Such patients as a rule, but not always, have EEG abnormalities which are indicative of temporal-lobe dysfunction.

Psychiatric Disorders of Epilepsy

Such disorders can be divided into three categories, as first suggested by Pond (1957). This subdivision consists of:

1. Disorders due to brain disease causing the fits
2. Disorders directly related to the seizures
3. Interictal disorders, which are unrelated in time to the occurrence of the seizures

As appears from reviews by Fenton (1981) and Bolwig (1986), the most interesting of these categories are the phenomena related to seizures and those representing interictal disorders.

Epilepsy is very often found in disorders due to brain disease, and it is well-known that both tumors and other localized brain lesions can cause focal brain syndromes that may be explained by changes in the frontal, temporal, occipital, or parietal lobes. A multitude of psychiatric phenomena represent the initial symptom of such a lesion, and cognitive, emotional, behavioural, and personality disorders can be observed in such cases. These disturbances have been comprehensively described by Lishman (1978). Disturbances of mental functioning are also very frequent, in diffuse cerebral disease with global intellectual impairment, the prevalence increasing with the severity of mental deficit (Corbett et al. 1975). Epileptic seizures are often observed in other organic brain syndromes, such as presenile dementia of the Alzheimer type or multiinfarct dementia.

The epileptic seizures probably representing an underlying brain pathology of hitherto unknown origin which are seen in many forms of psychosis in childhood have not so far been elucidated, but they point strongly to an organic background for psychoses such as infantile autism, atypical childhood psychosis, and some of the disintegrative forms of psychosis; for a review, see Fenton 1981.

Phenomena Related to Seizures

These are divided into preictal, ictal, and postictal events. The most important psychiatric disturbances directly connected to seizure activity are seen in complex partial seizures (CPS), psychomotor, and petit mal attacks. The term complex is used, because organized cerebral activity at a high level is affected, and the manifestations comprise a number of complex psychological phenomena such as changes in memory, ideation, and affect, illusions and hallucinations, as well as automatic behaviour (Gastaut and Broughton 1972). CPS probably occur due to a lesion in a particular part ofthe brain, and are usually of temporal lobe origin. With the development of the seizure, pronounced changes in the content of consciousness can be observed, sometimes leading to lack of responsiveness, confusion, and amnesia. The hallucinations are often well-formed and, with repeated attacks, are constant. This is in contrast to what is observed in many other organic brain syndromes and in elementary partial seizures.

To the patient, these experiences often represent an intrusion on his stream of consciousness, and he can be an observer of the pathological events, a condition which Hughlings Jackson termed mental diplopia (Jackson 1931).

Table 1 which gives the international classification. CPS are described under the following six categories: impaired consciousness only; cognitive symptomatology; affective symptomatology; psychosensory symptomatology; "psychomotor" symptomatology; and, compound forms which are simultaneous or sequential occurrences of any of the above symptoms.

It is thus evident that almost any form of psychopathology can occur in relation to seizures, and may often give rise to diagnostic problems.

Impairment of consciousness and psychomotor symptomatology are classical phenomena, and among the cognitive symptoms, those that have to do with memory functions are frequent in the form of illusions of memory. These can be in the form of either déjà-vu, déjà entendu, or déjà vécu, while the opposite in the form of jamais-vu, jamais entendu, and jamais vécu are also typical dysmnestic seizure phenomena. The two categories are contrasting, as they represent illusions of familiarity and strangeness, respectively. The external object or internal event seems to be perceived normally, but is poorly understood; Gastaut (1973) called this a nonperceptive or agnosic illusion.

Feelings of depersonalization and derealization-phenomena which also should be regarded as agnosic illusions are likewise well known.

Interictal Disorders

These are probably the most interesting phenomena for the psychiatrist, and they also represent the greatest problems in the process of diagnosing behavioural disorders. Recent studies pointing to an increased psychiatric morbidity in patients with epilepsy have been summarized by Trimble (1981). Most investigations made over the past 20 years indicate a higher incidence of abnormality in patients suffering from temporal-lobe epilepsy, in contrast to those with generalized seizures (Toone 1981). The most important interictal disturbances are various forms of personality disorder and psychoses, including affective disorders.

Psychosis and Epilepsy

The relationship between these conditions has been the subject of much discussion. There are descriptions dating back to Willis in the seventeenth century of the phenomenology of the chronic interictal psychoses. Since then, many psychiatrists have discussed the relationship between epilepsy and psychosis, especially Falret (1854), who introduced the terms periictal, interictal, and long-term insanity into this classification. The conditions in question are characterized by preserved clarity of consciousness. They can be affective, paranoid, or schizophrenia-like, with affective and schizo-affective symptomatology occurring most commonly. There seems to be a tendency in this category of patients for an intermittency in symptoms, with a recurrent course (Perez and Trimble 1980), while the schizophrenia-like or paranoid psychoses have a more chronic course. Toone (1981) gives a comprehensive review of the literature; it appears that patients with temporal-lobe epilepsy present the severest psychiatric problems (Table 2).

Although there are still numerous unanswered questions in connection with the psychiatric aspects of epilepsy, both experimental work and clinical observation point to the importance of the limbic system for development of psychopathology.

Interictal Personality Changes

This aspect of epilepsy is a widely debated issue. Some researchers, e.g., Stevens (1986) do not find any evidence of personality changes peculiar to epilepsy in patients with many years of epileptic manifestation, whereas others, especially Bear and Fedio (1977) and Waxman and Geschwind (1975), have described specific changes, including (a) change in sexuality, (b) hypermoralism, and (c) hypergraphia. These features are reported very often to be found together with lack of a sense of humour, circumstantiality, and viscosity (prolongation of social encounters).

This interictal personality syndrome is likely to be found especially in patients with CPS and a temporal EEG focus.

A recent review of the literature made by Sørensen and Bolwig (1987) finds that there is a raised prevalence of emotional and psychological problems in patients with epilepsy in general, and temporal-lobe epilepsy in particular.

Table 2. Salient characteristics of the interictal psychoses (from Toone 1981)

Authors	*n*	Type of psychoses[a]	Male: Female	Age of onset epilepsy	Age of onset psychosis	Interval	EEG	
							Temporal lobe foci (%)	Bilateral involvement (%)
Bartlett (1957)	11	M					72	
Slater et al. (1963)	69	S	46:33	15	30	15	80	25
Flor-Henry (1969)	50	M	26:24	13			*	44
Bruens (1971)	19	M	8:11	13	25	12	84	30
Taylor (1972)	13	M	5: 8					20
Jensen and Larsen (1979)	20	M		14	28	14	*	
Kristensen and Sindrup (1978a, b 1980)	96	P	46:50	12	34	22	*	30
Perez and Trimble (1980)	23	M	15: 8					
Toone and Driver (1980)	41	M						

* Selection limited to temporal-lobe epilepsy

[a] M, mixed; S, schizophrenia-like; P, paranoid

However, the existence of a specific behavioural syndrome of temporal-lobe epilepsy is not supported from the studies surveyed, although several case reports suggest a relationship between pronounced interest in philosophical/religious matters, hypergraphia, and altered sexuality – often hyposexuality.

Epilepsy, Neurophysiology, and Psychopathology

The renewed interest in epilepsy among psychiatrists comes partly from the availability of powerful modern means for the diagnosis of organic brain disease, especially that of focal origin, in psychiatric patients.

Apart from various forms of EEG measurement, including computer analysis of the architecture of electrical activity from both surface and deep electrodes, the most important recent techniques enable measurement of regional cerebral blood flow (rCBF) and brain metabolism in the form of positron emission tomography (PET). These have brought a new dimension to psychiatry, allowing the estimation of subtle changes in regional activity, and thereby opening up new possibilities in the process of diagnosing psychiatric illness. The findings in epilepsy by Ingvar (1975), Mazziotta and Engel (1984), and Trimble et al. (1984) point to a sophisticated elucidation of organic problems related to psychopathology.

The epilepsies, with their various psychiatric manifestations, may thus serve as an important model for studying gross psychopathology. With the new techniques mentioned above, not only can the electrical activity in the cerebral cortex be studied, but also the metabolic events taking place at various levels of the brain. Far greater possibilities than were available previously to classify the psychiatric disturbances of epilepsy therefore now exist.

With recent advances in molecular biology, genetics, and brain physiology a number of conditions previously described as "functional" may now be looked upon differently. The combination of studies of electrical and metabolic mapping of the brain with progress in molecular biology promises not only a better understanding of such illness, but also the possibility of making more accurate prognoses. With the present status of these new techniques, the epilepsies may probably serve as the best models for a general understanding of psychopathology.

Along with studies in human subjects suffering from epilepsy associated with mental disturbances, experimental studies in animals probably represent the best possibility of creating a link between neurophysiological disorder and psychopathology. In the laboratory, it is possible to look at well-controlled experiments in which discrete regions of the brain undergo some kind of influence leading to a abnormal behaviour, though, of course, in laboratory animals, psychopathology cannot be studied. Over the past two decades, various research groups have studied the "kindling" phenomenon, both in relation to epilepsy and to many other clinical conditions in humans, such as addiction, memory problems, and aggressive behaviour. The kindling model of epilepsy has recently been described by Goddard (1983), who was the first to point to this phenomenon in 1969 (Goddard et al. 1969). Experiments have shown that rats depleted of cerebral noradrenaline and therefore prone to kindling epilepsy normalize after intracerebral grafting of noradrenaline-rich cell suspensions from fetal locus coeruleus (Barry et al. 1987).

Thus, epilepsy represents one of the best situations available so far in which animal experiments and clinical-neurophysiological studies can be combined. These may possibly lead to a better understanding both of basic mechanisms of behaviour and of the psychopathology represented in the functional psychoses. With increased knowledge of the basic mechanisms underlying behaviour disorders, we may expect, say, within the next ten years, to see major revisions of the existing systems of classification of psychiatric illness. This will involve the addition of a neurobiological dimension, which today is only just becoming visible.

References

Barry DI, Kikvadze I, Brundin P, Bolwig TG, Björklund A, Lindvall O (1987) Grafted noradrenergic neurons suppress seizure development in kindling-induced epilepsy. Proc Natl Acad Sci USA 84:8712–8715

Bear DM, Fedio P (1977) Quantitative analysis of interictal behavior in temporal lobe epilepsy. Arch Neurol 34:454–457

Blumer D (ed) (1984) Psychiatric aspects of epilepsy. American Psychiatric Press, Washington

Bolwig TG (1986) Classification of psychiatric disturbances in epilepsy. In: Trimble MR, Bolwig TG (eds) Aspects of epilepsy and psychiatry. Wiley, Chichester, pp 1–8

Charcot JM (1877) Lectures on the diseases of the nervous system (transl. G. Sigerson). New Sydenham Society, London

Corbett JA, Harris R, Robinson RC (1975) Epilepsy. In: Wortis J (ed) Mental retardation and development disabilities, vol 7. Springer, Berlin Heidelberg New York, pp 79–111

Falret JP (1854) Mémoire sur la folie circulaire. Bulletin de l'Académie Imperiale de Médicine (Paris) 19:382–400

Fenton GW (1981) Psychiatric disorders of epilepsy: classification and phenomenology. In: Reynolds EH, Trimble MR (eds) Epilepsy and psychiatry. Churchill Livingstone, Edinburgh, pp 12–26

Freud S (1895) Studien über Hysterie. Deuticke, Leipzig

Gastaut H (1969) Clinical and electroencephalographical classification of epileptic seizures. Epilepsia [Suppl] 10:1–28

Gastaut H (1973) Dictionary of epilepsy. WHO, Geneva

Gastaut H, Broughton R (1972) Epileptic seizures. Springfield, Illinois

Goddard GV (1983) The kindling model of epilepsy. Trends Neurosci, July: 275–279

Goddard GV, McIntyre D, Leech C (1969) A permanent change in brain function resulting from daily electrical stimulations. Exp Neurol 25:295–330

Henderson D, Gillespie RD (1950) A textbook of psychiatry, 7th edn. Oxford University Press, London

Ingvar DH (1975) Regional CBF in focal cortical epilepsy. In: Langfitt TW, McHenry LC, Reivich M, Wollman H (eds) Cerebral circulation and metabolism. Springer, Berlin Heidelberg New York, pp 361–364

Jackson JH (1931) Selected writings of John Hughlings Jackson, vol 1. Hodder and Stroughton, London

Janet P (1907) The major symptoms of hysteria. Macmillan, London
Lishman WA (1978) Organic psychiatry. Blackwell Scientific, London
Littré E (ed) (1839–1861) Oeuvres complètes d'Hippocrate. vol 10. Baillière, Paris
Mazziotta JC, Engel J (1984) The use and impact of positron computed tomography scanning in epilepsy. Epilepsia 25 [Suppl 2]:84–104
Penfield W, Jasper HH (1954) Epilepsy and the functional anatomy of the human brain. Little Brown, Boston
Perez MM, Trimble MR (1980) Epileptic psychosis – diagnostic comparison with process schizophrenia. Br J Psychiatry 137:245–249
Pond DA (1957) Psychiatric aspects of epilepsy. J Indian Med Profession 3:1441–1451
Reynolds EH, Trimble MR (eds) (1981) Epilepsy and psychiatry. Churchill Livingstone, Edinburgh
Sørensen AS, Bolwig TG (1987) Personality and epilepsy: new evidence for a relationship? A review. Compr Psychiatry 28:369–383
Stevens JR (1986) Epilepsy and psychosis: neuropathological studies of six cases. In: Trimble MR, Bolwig TG (eds) Aspects of epilepsy and psychiatry. Wiley, Chichester, pp 117–145
Toone B (1981) Psychoses of epilepsy. In: Reynolds EH, Trimble MR (eds) Epilepsy and psychiatry. Churchill Livingstone, Edinburgh, pp 113–137
Trimble MR (1981) Neuropsychiatry. Wiley, Chichester
Trimble MR, Bolwig TG (eds) (1986) Aspects of epilepsy and psychiatry. Wiley, Chichester
Trimble MR, Bernardi S, Gallhofer B, Frackowiak RJS, Wise RJS, Jones T (1984) An interictal study of partial epilepsy using the oxygen-15 inhalation technique and positron emission tomography with special reference to psychosis. In: Baldy-Moulinier M, Ingvar DH, Meldrum BS (eds) Cerebral blood flow, metabolism and epilepsy. Libbey, London, pp 44–50
Waxman SG, Geschwind N (1975) The interictal behavior syndrome of temporal lobe epilepsy. Arch Gen Psychiatry 32:1580–1586

Epilepsy and Psychiatric Disorder

R. J. McClelland

> The epileptic neurosis is certainly most closely allied to the insane neurosis and when it exists in its masked form, affecting the mind for sometime before convulsions occur, it is hardly possible to distinguish it (Maudsley 1873).

The early reports of an association between psychiatric disorder and epilepsy were all based on biased samples, usually of psychiatric in-patients or psychiatric admissions (Slater et al. 1963). Studies of the relationship between specific forms of epilepsy, e.g. temporal lobe epilepsy and particular psychiatric syndromes, have again been restricted to specialist centres. It is not possible from such studies to establish the true rate or indeed the nature of the relationship between these two relatively common groups of disorders. There have been few detailed epidemiological studies in community-based samples (Pond and Bidwell 1960; Dowds et al. 1983; Toone 1986). Epidemiological investigations with larger samples are required, incorporating standardized rating scales to measure psychiatric morbidity and careful electro-clinical investigation.

Since relationship between epilepsy and psychiatric morbidity is frequently a complex one, epidemiological studies require to take into account both psychosocial and biological variables. For example, Rutter et al. (1970) have shown that children with epilepsy frequently have additional and interrelated social and psychological difficulties. Poor seizure control may have significant effects on schooling, which in turn may affect educational attainment, social adjustment, and peer relationships.

It is 25 years since Slater et al. (1963) first drew our attention to a possible link between temporal lobe epilepsy and an inter-ictal psychotic state, which was symptomatically identical to the schizophrenia group of disorders. Many studies since then have confirmed this finding. However, as Hill and Fenton (1969) have noted, despite the evidence in favour of an association between these two groups of disorders, the final answers regarding the magnitude and nature of the link must await detailed electro-clinical studies of random samples of patients with epilepsy. Is the schizophrenia associated with temporal lobe epilepsy simply a variant? Does temporal lobe epilepsy cause a release of the schizophrenic illness process? Present evidence would certainly suggest that the inter-ictal psychosis resembling schizophrenia occurs more often than chance in patients with temporal lobe epilepsy, and this association cannot be accounted for simply by the presence of temporal lobe pathology. In a small

Department of Mental Health, The Queen's University of Belfast, Whitla Medical Building, 97 Lisburn Road, Belfast BT9 7BL, Northern Ireland, UK

Interaction Between Mental and Physical Illness
Edited by R. Öhman et al.

number of patients, there would appear to be a relationship between seizure activity and psychosis. In some, seizure discharge leads to the appearance of the psychosis, while in others, psychotic manifestation is associated with a reduction in seizure frequency and in the EEG inter-ictal concomitants.

This link takes on greater significance with the renewed interest in the heterogeneity of schizophrenia. McGuffin et al. (1987), in their recent review of this issue, have concluded that no satisfactory link can be found between the different clinical typologies and genotype. The clinical exopheno-types are too remote from the underlying genetic expression (Gottesman and Shields 1972), so that phenotypal expression is more likely to be found at a physiological level within the brains of patients with schizophrenia. A closer understanding of the link between temporal lobe epilepsy and schizophrenia will almost certainly provide greater insight into the underlying pathophysiology of the schizophrenias and into the different contributions of genetic expression and acquired brain dysfunction in their causation.

The present focus at an anatomical or cellular level of organization for the pathogenesis of psychotic illness takes its origin from the concept of specific mental processes as unitary functions organized on a focal brain basis. Both these assumptions have recently been seriously questioned (Luria 1980; Miller 1986; Wexler 1986). The need to consider intermediate physiological processes seems essential to gaining a fuller understanding of the relationship between brain and mind. In such a model, specific behavior patterns, both normal and abnormal, are considered to arise at a higher level of organization than the cell, and are viewed as a final common path from a variety of alternative patterns of interactions between neural networks. The schizophreniform psychosis of temporal lobe epilepsy provides an important clinical example of the relationship between dysfunction within high-level physiological processes and psychopathology. The wide range of non-invasive methods which have recently become available for investigating cerebral function, embracing blood flow, metabolism, as well as brain electrical and magnetic field mapping and monitoring, provide new opportunities for investigating these high-level processes.

Perhaps a more profitable line of enquiry is to begin with temporal lobe dysfunction and examine its wider emotional and behavioural sequelae (Geschwind 1983). The neurophysiology of this disorder is well understood, and provides an almost unique clue to the links between altered brain function and behavioral change. These behavioral changes embrace transient states associated with the prodrome, the ictus, and the post-ictal phase. They also embrace the more enduring changes in personality and less commonly observed psychotic manifestations which are indistinguishable from schizophrenia itself.

One of the most intriguing forms of associations are the gradual personality changes observed with chronic temporal lobe epilepsy (Waxman and Geschwind 1975). Central within this syndrome is the development of intense concern with philosophical issues, a viscosity in thinking, and hypergraphia. These are often associated with irritability and hyposexuality. The contrasting features of the Kluver-Bucy syndrome, associated with lesions or disconnections of the temporal lobe, have led to the proposal of a hyperconnection model to account for the excessive investment of the environment with emotional significance produced by limbic excitation (Geschwind 1983; Bear 1979). Since stimulation of the limbic system can produce many of the observed behavioural associations of temporal lobe epilepsy, it is not surprising that spontaneous discharge within this system has similar effects. The propensity of mesial temporal lobe structures for kindling, i.e. becoming spontaneously active following infrequent stimulation, may provide a final common path for a variety of aetiological mechanisms which embrace both genetic loading and environmental insult.

The epileptic and behavioural sequelae of temporal lobe spiking may not always occur with equal frequency. Indeed, it is possible that the behavioural manifestations of temporal lobe spiking may occur in the absence of seizures. The implications of such an hypothesis are far-reaching for neuropsychiatry, and suggest a number of lines of enquiry: in-depth monitoring of patients with post-ictal and inter-ictal psychoses; epidemiological and electrophysiological studies of the hyperconnection syndrome; investigation of the different roles of psychotropic drugs and anticonvulsants in temporal lobe epilepsy, and the associated behavioural syndromes. In addition to human studies, it should also be possible to extend this work to animal investigation, permitting a more detailed study of the origin, locus, and distribution of the spike focus.

For over 100 years, clinicians and investigators have speculated on the relationship between epilepsy and psychiatric disorder, but until quite recently, it has not been possible to tease out these relationships. Only in the past few decades have coherent theories of brain functioning been advanced and subjected to the rigours of scientific investigation. During this period, the neural substrate for many aspects of higher functioning has been successfully elaborated. The recent emergence of monitoring and imaging techniques brings us to the threshold of a new era for the study of brain-behaviour relationships.

References

Bear DM (1979) Temporal lobe epilepsy – a syndrome of sensory-limbic hyperconnection. Cortex 15:357–384

Dowds N, McCluggage J, Nelson J (1983) A survey of the socio-medical aspects of epilepsy in a general practice population in Northern Ireland. British Epilepsy Association, London

Geschwind N (1983) Pathogenesis of behaviour change in temporal lobe epilepsy. In: Ward AA Jr, Perry JK, Purpura D (eds) Epilepsy. Raven New York, pp 355–370

Gottesman I, Shields J (1972) Schizophrenia a twin study vantage point. Academic, London

Hill D, Fenton GW (1969) The temporal lobe: EEG and disorders of behaviour. In: Herrington RN (ed) Current problems in neuropsychiatry. (British Journal of Psychiatry Special Publication No 4) Headley, Ashford, Kent, UK, pp 49–54

Luria AR (1980) Higher cortical functions in man, 2nd edn. Basic Books, New York
Maudsley H (1873) Body and mind, 2nd edn. Macmillan, London
McGuffin P, Farmer A, Gottesman II (1987) Is there really a split in schizophrenia? The genetic evidence. Br J Psychiatry 150:581–592
Miller L (1986) Narrow localizationism in psychiatric neuropsychology. Psychol Med 16:729–734
Pond DA, Bidwell BH (1960) A survey of epilepsy in 14 general practices. II Social and psychological aspects. Epilepsia 1:285–299
Rutter M, Graham PJ, Yule W (1970) A neuropsychiatric study in childhood. Clinics in developmental medicine. Heinemann, London
Slater E, Beard AW, Glithero E (1963) The schizophrenia-like psychosis of epilepsy. Br J Psychiatry 109:95–112
Toone B (1986) Epilepsy with mental illness: interrelationship. In: Trimble MR, Reynolds EH (eds) What is epilepsy? The clinical and scientific basis of epilepsy. Churchill Livingstone, London, pp 206–216
Waxman SG, Geschwind N (1975) The interictal behaviour syndrome of temporal lobe epilepsy. Arch Gen Psychiatry 32:1580–1586
Wexler B (1986) A model of brain function: its implications for psychiatric research. Br J Psychiatry 109:95–112

Physical Morbidity and Mortality in Psychiatric Patients

H. Häfner and H. Bickel

The risks of mortality and morbidity in mental patients are of interest in several respects. First, they may point to etiological links between mental disorders and physical illness. Second, they may have implications for treatment, and provide clues for preventive measures. In so far as they are not accounted for by selection mechanisms at the point of access to psychiatric treatment, mental illnesses may be associated in three different ways with increased or reduced risks for physical morbidity and mortality:

1. Through a direct relationship, emanating from psychiatric illness, which is the case, for example, in alcohol-related diseases or in depressive disorders with an elevated risk for suicide
2. Through an indirect relationship, mediated by factors associated with the mental disorder, such as deficient health behavior, self-neglect and immobility or long-term hospitalization as a protective factor against certain risks
3. Relationships between physical morbidity, mortality, and mental disorder may point to common underlying factors, e.g., coronary heart disease in conjunction with cerebrovascular dementia pointing to arteriosclerosis as a common basic disease, and this, in turn, to risk factors like hypertension and diabetes

The great variety of relevant factors associated both with mental disorder and physical illness, together with the complexity of their interaction, illustrate the scope of this topic and the considerable methodological problems involved. In studying these relationships, therefore, one first tries to find out whether the patterns of morbidity and mortality of the mentally ill differ in size and nature from those of the comparable general population. Since only a few studies have directly investigated the general and specific morbidity risks in mental patients, this review must be restricted to a much more widely and minutely studied mortality risk.

Zentralinstitut für Seelische Gesundheit J5, Postfach 122120, D-6800 Mannheim 1

Interaction Between Mental and Physical Illness
Edited by R. Öhman et al.

Psychiatric Disorders and Mortality Risk

Research Strategies

Since the first half of the last century, attempts to investigate the general mortality risk in psychiatric patients have been made in a large number of studies, applying a variety of methodological approaches (for a review see Alström 1942). Investigations restricted to cases of death in mental hospitals (Alström 1942; Ödegård 1936, 1951, 1952, 1967; Malzberg 1953; Larsson and Sjögren 1954) have the longest tradition; these provide a temporal cross-section of mortality during hospitalization. With the abandonment of custodial care and the expansion of active treatment, rehabilitation, and desinstitutionalization, it has become very questionable whether the remaining mental hospital patients can be regarded as representative for the total of treated psychiatric morbidity.

Against this backcloth, mortality research has undergone an increased differentiation in the past two decades. Results have been obtained at various levels of care, taking account of inpatients, outpatients, and discharged patients, as well as the total psychiatric morbidity, as identified in field studies, in a few cases. These studies have mainly employed two research strategies, which allow a longitudinal assessment of the mortality risk in patient cohorts, i.e., register-linkage studies and direct follow-up studies.

Register-linkage studies have the advantage of permitting the investigation of large patient samples. Since a patient is usually assumed to be alive unless his death is recorded, these studies have the disadvantage of probably underestimating the true mortality risk of a considerable degree because of erroneous or incomplete registration, which is primarily due to migration of patients.

Follow-up studies have the advantage of permitting a more detailed and reliable description of the patient cohort under study than do case register data. Another advantage is that the results are less liable to contain errors, as at anytime it can be checked whether a patient is still alive or not. A disadvantage is the amount of effort and expenditure required, which usually makes it impossible to use the sample sizes necessary for the testing of differential hypotheses.

In studies attempting to quantify the mortality risk in psychiatric patients, an identical methodology is used, irrespective of differences in research strategies, sample compositions, and lengths of observation periods. Since multivariate statistical devices for the analysis of survival times have only been available for a couple of years, subsamples were generally identified according to age, sex, and diagnostic groups, while both total mortality and mortality from specific causes has been related to the mortality in the general population. The quotient of observed and expected mortality, i.e., the "standard mortality ratio" (SMR), thus refers to the age- and sex-adjusted mortality risk of patients under study.

General Mortality Risk

Table 1 depicts some of the findings on mortality in psychiatric patients, compared with the general population, as obtained in large-scale studies in the past three decades.

The mortality risk in psychiatric inpatients has recently been assessed to be about three times the rate of the general population (Tokuhata and Stehman 1958; Saugstad and Ödegård 1979; Craig and Lin 1981). Studies that are based on a patient census which also includes discharged patients report an increase in risk by about twice only (Eastwood et al. 1982; Haugland et al. 1983; Wood et al. 1985; Martin et al. 1985a). The risk in various populations covering the

Table 1. Mortality of psychiatric patients in relation to the general population

Study	Sample	Risk period	Age of sample	Mortality ratio	
				Men	Women
Tokuhata and Stehman (1958)	Resident patients of mental hospitals, Michigan, U.S.A.	1950–1954	Age groups All ages	2.7–10.9 3.6	2.5–17.4 3.6
Babigian and Odoroff (1969)	Case register, Monroe County, N.Y., U.S.A.; $n=36529$	1960–1966	Age groups All ages	1.6– 3.2 2.5	0.4– 3.6 2.9
Innes and Millar (1970)	Psychiatric referrals, Scotland; $n=2103$	1960–1965	Age groups All ages	1.2– 6.8 1.8	1.4– 6.1 2.2
Rorsman (1974)	Mostly non-psychotic outpatients, Lund, Sweden; $n=3623$	1962–1968	Age groups All ages	1.0– 8.0 1.8	0.6– 7.7 1.4
Giel et al. (1978)	Long-stay patients in Dutch mental hospitals; $n=17211$	1970–1971	Age groups All ages	1.1– 9.3 1.7	1.2–21.0 1.8
Saugstad and Ödegård (1979)	Resident patients of mental hospitals, Norway	1969–1974	Age groups All ages	2.0– 5.5 2.4	3.1–15.3 3.5
Craig and Lin (1981)	Inpatients, state hospital, N.Y., U.S.A.	1969–1977	Age groups All ages	2.1– 5.9 2.6	2.6–14.0 3.3
Eastwood et al. (1982)	First admissions, Toronto, Canada; $n=1436$	1969–1978	Age groups All ages	1.0– 3.2 1.4	0.8– 8.7 1.6
Haugland et al. (1983)	Inpatients in 1975 or 1976, N.Y., U.S.A.; $n=1033$	1975–1978	Age groups All ages	1.8– 4.0 2.3	2.0– 4.4 2.2
Wood et al. (1985)	Current or former inpatients, Missouri, U.S.A.; 5268 deaths	1972–1976	Age groups All ages	1.0– 2.2 1.5	1.2– 2.4 1.7
Brook (1985)	Long-stay patients in Dutch mental hospitals; $n=12139$	1980–1981	Age groups All ages	1.3– 8.0 1.7	1.5–18.7 1.9

entire spectrum of treated psychiatric morbidity (Babigian and Odoroff 1969; Innes and Millar 1970) has been reported to be similar. As far as a comparison can be made, the findings of these studies are remarkably consistent and confirm a correlation between relative mortality, on the one hand, and age, sex, duration of illness, psychiatric diagnosis, and cause of death, on the other.

The age- and sex-specific life expectancy of the general population is levelled off in psychiatric patients. As Table 1 shows, there are considerable differences between the various age groups, with the size of the mortality risk ranging from one equal to that of the general population to one 20 times higher. The relative risks are usually highest in the youngest age groups and lowest for the oldest patients. Sex has a similar effect: the absolute mortality in female patients is not increased, compared with that in male patients, but their relative risk is generally increased, due to the higher life expectancy of females. These associations are consistent over the main diagnostic groups.

Cause-specific mortality in mental patients varies to different extents according to age, sex, and diagnosis; it has shown a reduction in "natural" mortality and an increase in "unnatural" causes of death in the course of the past few decades. This increased mortality seems to include all causes of death except malignant neoplasms. Although its proportion in the total mortality is low, the relative risk of dying from an infectious disease in a psychiatric hospital is still increased in the countries investigated (Saugstad and Ödegård 1979; Haugland et al. 1983; Wood et al. 1985).

Starting from diagnostic groups, symptomatic and organic psychoses show a strikingly high mortality risk, the lowest risk being found in functional psychiatric disorders and the greatest risk in the initial phase of an illness or at the beginning of treatment. In the first year of an inpatient treatment, the mortality rates were up to three times higher than in subsequent years (Craig and Lin 1981), whereas in long-stay patients (in hospital for more than two years), the mortality risk was increased by only 70%–90% (Giel et al. 1978; Brook 1985).

This led to the assumption that preexisting somatic diseases or risk factors may have increased the probability of psychiatric inpatient treatment. To eliminate this selection factor, mortality associated with psychiatric disorders was also investigated in field studies among unselected samples, but most of these studies were on elderly patients, and therefore permit only limited comparisons with the total of treated morbidity. The findings of these studies for elderly people were similar: psychoorganic disorders were also accompanied by a marked reduction of life expectancy in the general population (Kay and Bergmann 1966; Gilmore 1975; Nielsen et al. 1977; Magnusson and Helgason 1981; Bickel 1987), but with respect to functional psychiatric disorders, the correlation was less distinct. Whereas in some studies no excess mortality was found (Nielsen et al. 1977; Rorsman et al. 1982), Kay and Bergmann (1966), Persson (1981), and Enzell (1984) report an increased mortality risk. A multivariate study, in which further indicators influencing life expectancy were controlled, actually revealed that further life expectancy was reduced by half (Bickel 1987).

Compared with studies of psychiatric patients, the few field studies also or exclusively focussing on young persons found the natural mortality risk to be less markedly increased; this can partly be explained by the lower severity of the mental disorders encountered in the community. The Lundby Study also revealed the mortality risk to be significantly increased in severe disorders requiring psychiatric treatment (Rorsman et al. 1983). In addition, field studies have shown the mortality risk to be elevated in conjunction with organic brain syndromes (Rorsman et al. 1985), alcohol abuse (Halldin et al. 1985) and depressive disorders (Murphy et al. 1987). In the Stirling County Study, affective disorders were demonstrated to be more closely associated with further life expectancy than are physical diseases. Only in the Midtown Manhattan Restudy (Singer et al. 1976) was the mean life expectancy of the mentality impaired equal to that of mentally healthy individuals. This may probably be explained by the employment of a relatively wide definition of psychological impairment in the study, but mentally ill individuals died from cardiovascular or cerebrovascular and alcohol-related diseases and became victims of violent death more often than mentally healthy persons.

Disease-Specific Risks of Natural Causes of Death

In treated patients systematic covariations can be observed between the mortality risk and psychiatric diagnoses, causes of death, and demographic indicators; therefore, the findings are confounded by differences in the composition of samples. Conclusions as to whether death risks are diagnosis-specific or cause-specific can therefore be drawn only from homogeneous samples.

In schizophrenia, the death risk has been assessed with a high degree of consistency. In the first half of this century, when schizophrenics accounted for two-thirds of mental inpatients, this risk was characterized by a high mortality from tuberculosis during stay in hospital (Alström 1942; Ödegård 1952), but with the eradication of tuberculosis in these hospitals, the mortality risk in schizophrenia decreased markedly. As Table 2 shows, both for males and females, it is almost twice as high as in the general population; in the past few decades, this situation has not changed essentially, and at present, the risk in nonhospitalized patients seems to equal that in the hospitalized. The risk is increased particularly in younger age groups and in the initial phase of the disease (Black et al. 1985c), but with advancing years, the life expectancy of schizophrenics approximates that of the general population (Herrman et al. 1983; Allebeck and Wistedt 1986). Insofar as the increased mortality could not be ascribed exclusively to unnatural causes (Black et al. 1985c), it was apparently nonspecific (Allebeck and Wistedt 1986), most likely pointing to an accumulation of cardiovascular diseases (Hermann et al. 1983; Saugstad and Ödegård 1985). Though the explanations of increased mortality are divergent, none assume an inherent biological disadvantage, but rather refer to changes in lifestyle and environmental conditions. Amdur and Souchek (1981) have

Table 2. Mortality of schizophrenic patients in relation to the general population

Study	Sample	Risk period	Mortality ratio	
			Men	Women
Malzberg (1953)	First admissions, New York, U.S.A.; $n=5901$	1943–1948	1.8	2.0
Babigian and Odoroff (1969)	Case register Monroe County, U.S.A.	1960–1966	1.6	1.9
Giel et al. (1978)	Long-stay patients in Dutch mental hospitals; $n=8142$	1970–1971	1.2	1.1
Saugstad and Ödegård (1979)	Resident patients mental hospitals, Norway	1969–1974	2.0	2.3
Müller (1981)	Inpatients before 1963, Lausanne, Switz.	Until age off 65+	1.6	1.8
Eastwood et al. (1982)	First admissions, Toronto, Canada	1969–1978	1.0	2.2
Herrman et al. (1983)	Case register, Oxfordshire, U.K.; $n=592$	1971–1977	2.0	1.9
Haugland et al. (1983)	Inpatients, Rockland County, U.S.A.	1975–1978	2.1	1.6
Wood et al. (1985)	Resident patients of mental hospitals, Missouri, U.S.A.; $n=709$	1972–1976	1.5	1.2
Black et al. (1985c)	Former inpatients, Iowa, U.S.A.; $n=688$	1972–1981	2.4	2.8
Brook (1985)	Long-stay patients in Dutch mental hospitals; $n=5226$	1980–1981	1.6	1.6
Allebeck and Wistedt (1986)	Discharged patients, Stockholm County, Sweden; $n=1190$	1971–1981	2.3	2.5
Kendler (1986)	Twin register, Veterans Adm., U.S.A.; $n=590$	1946–1981	1.8	–

verified the essential influence of alcohol abuse in schizophrenic outpatients, while Saugstad and Ödegård (1985) assume that the side-effects of medication which cause low activity and weight gain may increase the risk of cardiovascular diseases. Selection effects have been indirectly evaluated by Hermann et al. (1983), who compared the number of recorded hospital admissions of schizophrenic patients for physical diseases with the figures expected for the general population: although they observed an increased natural mortality, the increase in utilization was ascertained to be due only to the sequelae of accidents or attempted suicides. They consider a schizophrenia-specific physical morbidity risk to be improbable, as does Kendler (1986), who conducted an extensive twin study.

For affective disorders, excess mortality, especially in male patients, is reported to amount to up to four times the rates of the general population (Kerr et al. 1969; Haughland et al. 1983).

Presumably because of differences in the composition of the populations investigated and the low reliability of diagnosis, the variance between these empirical findings was greater than in schizophrenia. On average, the mortality risk seems to be lower, and primarily attributable to unnatural causes (Black et al. 1985c), while a decline in excess mortality has also become apparent over recent decades (Tsuang and Simpson 1985). Once again, the risk is increased in younger age groups and in the first years following the onset of affective disorders (Black et al. 1985c). There are no indications of associations with natural causes of death, the risk of cancer, in particular, seeming not to be increased (Tsuang et al. 1980). The most striking result is reported by Martin et al. (1985b), who attribute the entire excess risk to secondary affective disorders, whereas in primary affective disorders, they did not find the risk to be elevated. However, in view of the small size of the sample and the few death cases investigated, this result only underlines the importance of diagnostic differentiation before the finding can be definitely confirmed.

In severe neuroses, too, the mortality risk seems to be increased by 50%–100% (Babigian and Odoroff 1969; Sims and Prior 1978; Coryell et al. 1982; Black et al. 1985c; Brook 1985). But the definition of this diagnostic group is too imprecise to allow exact comparisons. Sims (1978), who has reexamined the largest sample of treated neurotic patients over a lengthy period of time, came to the conclusion that even after subtracting the unnatural causes of death, the risk was increased by 60%. He assumed that somatic diseases which the patients might suffer from when treated for neurosis did not account for this risk; this was because every patient had been thoroughly examined, cases of death due to diseases known to produce neurotic symptoms did not occur, and the risk did not rise in the first year after discharge, but only over the course of time. On the other hand, he suggested that neurotics might be far more exposed to well-known risks such as alcohol and nicotine abuse, might be more susceptible to somatic diseases in the future, and that intercurrent diseases in them might take a more unfavourable course. Other studies of neurotic patients have replicated the widely known pattern of an elevated initial mortality, and have found causes of violent death to rank highest (Black et al. 1985c). Coryell et al. (1982) assume the increased risk to be attributable primarily to "panic disorders."

An essential risk factor of mortality among psychiatric patients is to be seen in the effects of behavior that is harmful to health. Longitudinal studies report a mortality rate of up to 21% for anorexia nervosa (Hsu 1980; Steinhausen and Glanville 1983) as a direct sequelae of the disorder. In alcohol abuse, the association is similarly distinct, the mean mortality risk in treated alcohol addicts being two or three times the rate of the general population (Schmidt and de Lint 1969); it is particularly high in younger patients and in females (Taylor et al. 1983). The mortality risk can be attributed almost entirely to alcohol-related and violent causes of death, which account for the excess mortality almost equally (Berglund 1984; Berglund and Tunving 1985).

Among the causes of natural death, cirrhosis of the liver and cardiovascular and gastrointestinal diseases predominate, whereas suicides prevail in the causes of violent deaths. In addition, there is some indication that alcohol also plays a decisive role in excess mortality among other diagnostic groups: Babigian and Odoroff (1969) have observed a considerable increase in the mortality risk, especially among females, when alcohol abuse was diagnosed at the same time. In the study by Amdur and Souchek (1981), the mortality risk increased threefold when alcohol or drug abuse occurred in the patients' past history. It therefore seems necessary to consider the consumption of alcohol, which is associated with psychiatric disorders and abnormal behavior, as a mediating factor for physical morbidity and mortality.

In recent years, mortality has been investigated more thoroughly in the mentally retarded than that in any other group of mental disorders. The findings can be summarized as follows: as a result of education, better nutrition, reduction in the risks of infection, and successful control of concurrent diseases, life expectancy has increased drastically by 30 to 40 years from 1930 to 1980 – as was shown by Carter and Jancar (1983) for a hospital population. From a Scottish study among mentally retarded who had already reached the age of 45, Tait (1983) deduced that their future life expectancy was similar to that of the general population.

Nevertheless, the morbidity risk is still markedly increased during the first years of life in the case of mental retardation. A comprehensive Finnish cohort study (Similae et al. 1986) covering the period from birth up to the age of 16, showed that the mean mortality in the mentally retarded was seven times the level of the general population. The risk rose parallel to the degree of severity of retardation, and was primarily determined by the basic etiology and the malformations associated with it. This early mortality is particularly marked in those 20%–40% of the mentally retarded with Down's syndrome who suffer from a congenital heart disease (Fryers 1986).

Whereas studies in the 1940s and 1950s reported that only 40%–50% of individuals suffering from Down's syndrome survived to the age of 5 years, the rate now varies between 77% and 87% (Fryers 1986). As shown in a nationwide Danish study of approximately 2500 patients, their life expectancy runs parallel to that of the general population (Dupont et al. 1986b), though it is equal in both sexes and reduced by 10 to 20 years at any point in time. After exogenic risks have largely been ruled out, this pattern of mortality raises the question whether the "natural" lifespan is shortened in Down's syndrome. The hypothesis of premature ageing opens up interesting aspects of research, which have already received a great deal of attention in connection with the etiological association with senile dementia of the Alzheimer type, by way of a gene on chromosome no. 21 (Heston et al. 1981; Cutler et al. 1985; Kang et al. 1987).

In the heterogeneous category of symptomatic and organic psychoses, mortality is highly increased, but unnatural causes of death are of secondary importance. The age-standardized risk is particularly high in younger patients, indicating a high proportion of severe diseases or traumata of the brain as underlying causes for their mental conditions. However, in the majority of these studies, diagnostic differentiation is insufficient and the number of younger patients too small to allow useful comparisons (Black et al. 1985b).

Because of the growing number of mentally impaired elderly people and the increased public interest in the health and mortality risks of the aged, the mortality risk in this diagnostic group of symptomatic and organic psychoses has been investigated primarily among elderly patients. Thirty years ago, Roth (1955) had already stated that the natural course of organic mental disorders in old age is characterized by high mortality. In recent decades, the mean death rate of patients with dementia who had been admitted to hospital amounted to 40% after 1 year, to 60% after 2 years, and reached 80% after 5 years. A study including nearly 1000 demented patients in Geneva (Go et al. 1978) has revealed that after the onset of the disease, their life expectancy was three-tenths, and after hospital admission as low as one-tenth of the general life expectancy in persons of the same age. Various studies have shown the remaining life expectancy of patients with these psychoses to be considered reduced even when statistically controlled for age, sex, and physical handicaps (Jarvik et al. 1980; Vitalino et al. 1981; Campbell et al. 1985; Bickel 1987). In fact, the survival time of such patients seems to be independent of their age. This also emphasizes that underlying pathological processes effect a course of dementia which is limited in time and ends in death, and that cognitive impairment is not a simple concomitant phenomenon of physiological ageing. Independent of age at the onset of the disease, the mean survival time with these diagnoses ranges from 6 to 8 years (Heston 1981; Barclay et al. 1985; Mölsä et al. 1986; Diesfeldt et al. 1986).

There are, however, characteristic differences between the primarily degenerative types of presenile and senile dementia, e.g., Alzheimer's disease, and the cerebrovascular types like multiinfarct dementia. Whereas life expectancy in Alzheimer's dementia is closely related to the severity of cognitive impairment, and indicates that the disease is a process (Nielsen et al. 1977; Mölsä et al. 1986), survival times in multiinfarct dementia do not display any systematic correlation with the degree of severity. Also, the mortality due to multiinfarct dementia has remained at a consistent level in the last decades, while there are increasing indications of lengthened survival times in Alzheimer's disease (Christie 1982, 1985; Christie and Train 1984; Blessed and Wilson 1982; Duckworth et al. 1979; Barclay et al. 1985; Rorsman et al. 1985). It is still an open question whether the causes of this difference are to be found in the successful control of concurrent lethal diseases or in a greater number of Alzheimer's cases following milder courses, for unknown reasons.

Should the life expectancy of patients with Alzheimer's disease and the duration of the disease actually have increased, the discovery of the responsible factors could contribute to a better understanding of this form of dementia. The same is true for the explanation of interindividual variance in the survival time. It has not yet been possible to identify any risk factor of prognostic relevance, except the degree of severity of brain dysfunction (Kaszniak et al. 1978; Katona et al. 1983).

Risk of Violent Death

According to some of the reported empirical findings, excess mortality in some of the diagnostic groups can be attributed largely or even entirely to the increased frequency of violent deaths, particularly from suicides and accidents. The ratio of deaths from these causes among psychiatric inpatients with functional disorders is 22% (Saugstad and Ödegård 1985). For discharged or outpatients, figures ranging from 28% to 48% have been reported (Forssman and Jannson 1960; Rorsman 1974; Amdur and Souchek 1981; Eastwood et al. 1982; Martin et al. 1985 b; Black et al. 1985 a; Ribourdouille and Corten 1986). In various diagnostic groups, the proportions of unnatural causes of death in total mortality are fairly similar. In affective disorders it is reported to vary between 26% and 31% (Coryell 1981; Eastwood et al. 1982; Black et al. 1985 c), in schizophrenia between 29% and 49% (Eastwood et al. 1982; Herrman et al. 1983; Black et al. 1985 c), and in alcohol abuse between 30% and 39% (Berglund 1984; Berglund and Tunving 1985; Black et al. 1985 c). The respective excess mortality calculated for unnatural causes of death reaches a maximum of 30 times the expected value (Innes and Millar 1970), and amounts to an average of about tenfold that of the general population.

Risk of Suicide

In recent times, suicide has played a decisive role among the various causes of increased mortality in psychiatric patients. Earlier a number of studies proved that in several European countries, the frequency of suicide during inpatient treatment and after discharge considerably increased, both absolutely and relatively; in some cases, it was even multiplied several times (Hessö 1977; Langley and Bayatti 1984; Perris et al. 1980; Ernst et al. 1980; Modestin 1982; Saugstad and Ödegård 1985). The first weeks following admission are the period of the most increased risk (Barner-Rasmussen 1986), though most of these suicides are not registered in the hospital statistics, since they are committed after discharge. Therefore, suicide figures calculated on this basis usually underestimate the risk in mental inpatients to a considerable extent. A nationwide study in Denmark showed that slightly over 20% commit suicide during hospital admission, but that nearly 80% do so in the first year after discharge (Barner-Rasmussen et al. 1986). Even the majority of the suicides occurring during inpatient treatment are committed outside hospital (Allebeck et al. 1986). According to case register studies, the overall suicide risk in psychiatric patients is ten times the rate of the general population (Babigian and Odoroff 1969). In follow-up studies of discharged patients, relative risks were found that amounted to 40 times the rate of the general population (Black et al. 1985 a).

It is primarily affective psychoses, alcohol- and drug-abuse, schizophrenia, and neuroses that seem to contribute to suicide mortality (Barner-Rasmussen et al. 1986). In affective psychoses, alcohol addiction, and drug abuse, the lifetime risk is estimated at 15%, and in schizophrenia at 10% (Hawton 1987). Follow-up studies have shown that excess mortality due to unnatural causes of death was increased by 5 to 13 times in male alcohol addicts, and by 6 to 25 times in females (Taylor et al. 1983; Eastwood et al. 1982; Berglund 1984; Berglund and Tunving 1985). Especially in younger age groups, drug abuse can be assumed to be associated with suicide (Benson and Holmberg 1984). Unnatural causes of death were found to be increased by 6 to 10 times in affective disorders (Tsuang 1978; Coryell 1981; Eastwood et al. 1982; Black et al. 1985c), in schizophrenia by 4 to 13 times (Tsuang 1978; Eastwood et al. 1982; Herrman et al. 1983; Black et al. 1985c; Allebeck and Wistedt 1986; Kendler 1986), and in neuroses by 4 to 8 times the rate of the general population (Coryell et al. 1982; Sims 1984; Black et al. 1985c). The reduction in the frequency of suicide seems to be the most obvious indication that premature deaths of psychiatric patients could be prevented: nearly all suicides included in the Lundby Study suffered from mental disorders (Hagnell et al. 1981). Due to the extension of mental health services in European countries, many more people than in the past receive psychiatric care (Shaw and Sims 1984). The Monroe County Register (Kraft and Babigian 1976) has revealed that about 50% of those who committed suicide had sought psychiatric help before doing so, but in spite of such extensive utilization, the suicide rates had not been reduced. In younger age groups or younger birth cohorts, the frequency of suicides seems to be markedly increasing in some countries (Canada, the USA, and Australia), to a lesser extent or only in some younger age groups in the FRG and Switzerland, and not at all in Sweden (Schmidtke and Häfner 1985). A more exact knowledge of the triggering and risk factors for suicide is therefore of the utmost importance (WHO 1986).

Physical Morbidity in Mental Disorders

The increased mortality in psychiatric patients finds its parallel in the quantitative association between psychiatric and somatic disorders, some of which have been sufficiently confirmed by epidemiological studies (Lipowsky 1975). In a survey of about a dozen studies conducted in the past 40 years, Koranyi (1980) draws the conclusion that about 50% of mental-hospital patients additionally suffer from somatic diseases. This high prevalence can be ascribed to a variety of causes.

One of the reasons is the fact that certain somatic diseases cause mental disorders: Hall et al. (1978) have examined psychiatric outpatients and came to the conclusion that in 9% of the cases, a somatic disease had caused the psychiatric symptoms. Endocrine, infectious, pulmonary, and gastrointestinal diseases were the most frequent medical disorders involved. The most frequent psychiatric disorders consisted in depressive and anxiety neuroses, reactive psychoses, schizophrenia, psychoorganic syndromes, and personality disorders. It was emphasized that the absence of specificity of the psychiatric symptoms made it difficult to separate the somatic from functional causes. In a further study of a hospital population (Hall et al. 1980), 46% of the somatic diseases diagnosed were asssumed to have caused or aggravated the psychiatric symptoms, while in 61% of the patients, the psychiatric symptoms quickly faded away after medical treatment.

A further direct risk may consist in the self-harming effects of abnormal behavior. Alcohol abuse, for example, increases the risk of carcinomas of the mouth, esophagus, stomach, and liver, the risk of heart disease and cirrhosis of the liver, as well as a weakening of the immune system. Drug abuse increases the probability of hepatitis and other severe infections, while insufficient fluid intake and eating owing to anorexia, depression, or dementia have serious, and sometimes fatal effects on the electrolyte metabolism.

Noncompliance due to psychiatric disorder may have an unfavorable impact on the course of persisting diseases such as diabetes mellitus. Measures for treating the psychiatric disorder may also entail further risks to health: the formerly high mortality in mental hospitals due to tuberculosis may serve as an example. Indications that the long-term intake of psychotropic drugs favors overweight and hypertension and consequently increases cardiac risks, need thorough examination (Schwalb et al. 1981; Gopalaswamy and Morgan 1985).

A further reason for the increased morbidity and mortality in mental patients may be found in selective factors. As a result of the additional strain caused by a somatic disease, psychiatric patients may be more ready to contact a mental health service, and may thus contribute to the increase in the somatically ill among psychiatric patients. Since not every psychiatric disorder is evenly distributed over all population groups, psychiatric patients might to a larger degree be afflicted with health risks, or might have been exposed to health risks which are not considered in the usual comparisons with morbidity and mortality in the general population.

Reduced Morbidity Risks in Mental Disorders

For a long time, researchers have been investigating the assumedly diminished risk of cancer in schizophrenia (Commissioners in Lunacy for England and Wales 1909). The conclusions have mainly been based on mortality studies in schizophrenia, which did not allow for the reduced life expectancy and the low mean age of schizophrenics at death. Some more recent studies have also shown the risk to be reduced, but their findings are not consistent. Only in the past few years have register-linkage studies, most of which have been coordinated by WHO, assessed the incidence of cancer in schizophrenic patients by means of an adequate methodological approach, and compared it with the rates in the general population. In the most comprehensive one, i.e., the Danish study covering 100000 person-years, the age-standardized incidence of all carcinomata was diminished by 33% in male and by 8% in female schizophrenics (Dupont et al. 1986a). Both in males and in females, the risk of lung cancer and of carcinoma of the prostate and the cervix uteri respectively was considerably reduced. However, since a series of relevant variables could not be controlled, the interpretation of the findings is difficult. The assumption of the authors that schizophrenia or the care provided for those with it may be associated with reduced environmental risks for carcinomas, for instance, with less cigarette smoking in males and less sexual intercourse in female schizophrenics, sounds plausible. An antitumor effect of neuroleptic drugs, which has not yet been confirmed, is also under investigation.

However, instead of a reduction in mortality, the Japanese part of the WHO project reported a significant increase of 50% (Nakane and Ohta 1986). The relative risk for breast cancer actually exceeded the expectation values by 220%, which might be a further indication of the unproven assumption that a rise in the prolactin level due to phenothiazine may have a carcinogetic effect.

Thus, the findings on a possibly protective effect of schizophrenia are inconsistent. Although there seems to be evidence for a reduced morbidity rate for rheumatic arthritis in schizophrenic patients, confirmation of this is still lacking (Baldwin 1979), and at present, there is no indication of the incidence of other physical diseases being reduced in mental disorders (Tsuang et al. 1983).

Conclusion

The considerably increased average mortality risk in psychiatric disorders that are not lethal in themselves and not determined by an underlying physical disease is a challenge for psychiatric research. Therefore, monitoring of trends in the mortality patterns of psychiatric patients by means of case register studies needs to be pursued in the long term. It is very regrettable that the use of disease registers and the indispensable research device of record linkage is hindered by restrictive data protection regulations. Answering questions in this important field of research almost invariably requires the investigation of large samples over long periods of time, which can only be accomplished with the help of effectively functioning registers. It is also necessary to be able to link personal data with death-register and morbidity (treatment or social security) data. In countries in which the establishment of new registers or the running of existing ones and record linkage are not permitted, legislators and public opinion should be educated in the necessity of these research devices and informed about the existing data protection and confidentiality regulations. In this way, the use of disease registers for research purposes could be rendered considerably more secure from misuse than the traditional records and case-notes.

Studies of mortality in mental patients, the majority of which have been conducted on the basis of register data, have yielded fairly consistent empirical evidence of some fundamental associations. They have shown that although the life expectancy of psychiatric patients has increased in the past few decades, these patients still have an excess risk for natural causes of death. This elevated mortality is not restricted to inpatients or to certain diagnostic groups. It can also be demonstrated in discharged and outpatients, in unselected samples in field studies, and in both functional psychoses and severe neuroses.

However, the evidence for specific associations between psychiatric diagnosis and natural causes of death is not yet conclusive. Cardiovascular causes of death rank first in quantitative terms, whereas the mortality risk for cancer shows the smallest deviation from expected values.

Morbidity risks in mental patients have so far been investigated mainly in cross-sectional studies, whose findings indicate that many of the mentally ill also suffer from somatic diseases. It has not been possible to prove conclusively that morbidity risks are reduced. Although some studies seem to point to reduced morbidity and mortality for cancer in schizophrenic patients, the results are still inconsistent and require further evaluation.

In younger age-groups in particular, and in patients treated for functional psychiatric disorders or alcohol and drug abuse, a large proportion of the observed excess mortality is accounted for by unnatural causes of death. Among these patients, suicide is by far the most frequent cause of premature death. Rates for suicides committed during inpatient treatment in mental hospital and after discharge or during outpatient treatment seem to have increased continuously for psychiatric patients in the past few decades.

To better understand the relationships between physical and mental disorders and to prevent premature deaths in psychiatric patients, it is therefore necessary to conduct studies that help to identify more reliably the risk factors contributing to increased mortality in these patients. Since it is to be assumed that a simultaneous presence of physical and mental disease exerts an unfavorable influence on the course of both, studies investigating interactions between diseases, e.g., depression and diabetes, seem promising. Because of the increasing ageing of the populations in industrial countries, it will be of increasing importance to obtain knowledge of the effects of psychogeriatric disorders on age-related physical diseases.

The elevated mortality in mental patients in the first 2 years after onset of the disorder or commencement of treatment poses the question whether preexisting physical morbidity either contributes to the onset of mental disorders or exacerbates them, or whether physical morbidity manifests itself for the first time when psychiatric symptoms are already present. In respect of the long-term course, it is of interest to know to what extent mediating factors such as concomitant depressive disorders, differing lifestyles, behavioral patterns relevant to health, and long-term treatment with psychotropic drugs prove detrimental to health. In this context, the question arises how these behavioral patterns can be changed in order to reduce health risks.

Finally, in view of increasing suicide figures, particularly in affective disorders, schizophrenia, and alcohol and drug abuse, research efforts must be multiplied to identify the risk factors more precisely and obtain clues for preventive action so that persons at risk can be protected better. From clinical studies, a number of risk factors have been described; their role must now be assessed in large-scale, and if possible prospective longitudinal studies.

Needed Areas of Research

1. Long-term monitoring of mortality risks in psychiatric patients by case register and linkage strategies: Recommendations that governments should guarantee the continuation of case or disease registers, with the observation of data protection regulations, in order to secure the protection of personal data
2. Prospective studies of sufficiently large samples to identify possible differences in morbidity risks in certain mental disorders (e.g., schizophrenia and the risk for carcinosis and rheumatic diseases)
3. Investigation of indirect risks for sequelae mediated by related forms of behavior (self-neglect, deficient coping strategies) or measures of treatment in psychiatric disorders, especially among the elderly
4. Search for risk factors accounting for the increased suicide rates in mental patients, as well as to assist approaches for preventive action

References

Allebeck P, Wistedt B (1986) Mortality in schizophrenia. A ten-year follow-up based on the Stockholm county inpatient register. Arch Gen Psychiatry 43:650–653

Allebeck P, Varla A, Wistedt B (1986) Suicide and violent death among patients with schizophrenia. Acta Psychiatr Scand 74:43–49

Alström CH (1942) Mortality in mental hospitals with especial regard to tuberculosis. Acta Psychiat Neurol Scand [Suppl] 24

Amdur MA, Souchek J (1981) Death in aftercare. Compr Psychiatry 22:619–626

Babigian HM, Odoroff CL (1969) The mortality experience of a population with psychiatric illness. Am J Psychiatry 126:470–480

Baldwin JA (1979) Schizophrenia and physical disease. Psychol Med 9:611–618

Barclay LL, Zemcov A, Blass JP, Sansone J (1985) Survival in Alzheimer's disease and vascular dementias. Neurology 35:834–840

Barner-Rasmussen P (1986) Suicide in psychiatric patients in Denmark, 1971–1981. II. Hospital utilization and risk groups. Acta Psychiatr Scand 73:449–455

Barner-Rasmussen P, Dupont A, Bille H (1986) Suicide in psychiatric patients in Denmark, 1971–81. I. Demographic and diagnostic description. Acta Psychiatr Scand 73:441–448

Benson G, Holmberg MB (1984) Drug-related mortality in young people. Acta Psychiatr Scand 70:525–534

Berglund M (1984) Mortality in alcoholics related to clinical state at first admission. Acta Psychiatr Scand 70:407–416

Berglund M, Tunving K (1985) Assaultive alcoholics 20 years later. Acta Psychiatr Scand 71:141–147

Bickel H (1987) Psychiatric illness and mortality among the elderly: findings of an epidemiological study. In: Cooper B (ed) Psychiatric epidemiology. Croom Helm, London, pp 192–211

Black DW, Warrack G, Winokur G (1985a) The Iowa record-linkage study. I. Suicide and accidental deaths among psychiatric patients. Arch Gen Psychiatry 42:71–75
Black DW, Warrack G, Winokur G (1985b) The Iowa record-linkage study. II. Excess mortality among patients with organic mental disorders. Arch Gen Psychiatry 42:78–81
Black DW, Warrack G, Winokur G (1985c) The Iowa record-linkage study. III. Excess mortality among patients with "functional" disorders. Arch Gen Psychiatry 42:82–88
Blessed G, Wilson ID (1982) The contemporary natural history of mental disorder in old age. Br J Psychiatry 141:59–67
Brook OH (1985) Mortality in the long-stay population of Dutch mental hospitals. Acta Psychiatr Scand 71:626–635
Campbell AJ, Diep C, Reinken J, McCosh L (1985) Factors predicting mortality in a total population sample of the elderly. J Epidemiol Community Health 39:337–342
Carter G, Jancar J (1983) Mortality in the mentally handicapped: a 50 year survey at the Stoke Park group of Hospitals (1930–1980). J Ment Defic Res 27:143–156
Christie AB (1982) Changing patterns in mental illness in the elderly. Br J Psychiatry 140:154–159
Christie AB (1985) Survival in dementia: a review. In: Arie T (ed) Recent advances in psychogeriatrics 1. Churchill Livingstone, Edinburgh, pp 33–43
Christie AB, Train JD (1984) Change in the pattern of care for the demented. Br J Psychiatry 144:9–15
Commissioners in Lunacy for England and Wales (1909) Annual Report. HMSO, London
Coryell W (1981) Diagnosis-specific mortality. Primary unipolar depression and Briquet's syndrome (somatization disorder). Arch Gen Psychiatry 38:939–942
Coryell W, Noyes R, Clancy J (1982) Excess mortality in panic disorder. A comparison with primary unipolar depression. Arch Gen Psychiatry 39:701–710
Craig TJ, Lin SP (1981) Mortality among psychiatric inpatients. Age-adjusted comparison of populations before and after psychotropic drug era. Arch Gen Psychiatry 38:935–938
Cutler NR, Heston LL, Davies P, Haxby JV, Shapiro MB (1985) Alzheimer's disease and Down's syndrome: new insights. Ann Intern Med 103:566–578
Diesfeldt HFA, van Houte LR, Moerkens RM (1986) Duration of survival in senile dementia. Acta Psychiatr Scand 73:366–371
Duckworth GS, Kedward HB, Bailey WF (1979) Prognosis of mental illness in old age. A four year follow-up study. Can J Psychiatry 24:674–682
Dupont A, Möller Jensen O, Strömgren E, Jablensky A (1986a) Incidence of cancer in patients diagnosed as schizophrenic in Denmark. In: ten Horn GHMM, Giel R, Gulbinat WH, Henderson JH (eds) Psychiatric case registers in public health. Elsevier, Amsterdam, pp 229–239
Dupont A, Væth M, Videbech P (1986b) Mortality and life expectancy of Down's syndrome in Denmark. J Ment Defic Res
Eastwood MR, Stiasny S, Meier HMR, Woogh CM (1982) Mental illness and mortality. Compr Psychiatry 23:377–385
Enzell K (1984) Mortality among persons with depressive symptoms and among responders and non-responders in a health check-up. An investigation of persons born in 1905 and followed up from age 66 to 75. Acta Psychiatr Scand 69:89–102
Ernst K, Moser U, Ernst C (1980) Zunehmende Suicide psychiatrischer Klinikpatienten: Realität oder Artefakt? Arch Psychiatr Nervenkr 228:351–363
Forssman H, Jansson B (1960) Follow-up study of 849 men admitted for mental disorders to the psychiatric ward of a general hospital. Acta Psychiatr Neurol Scand 35:57–72
Fryers T (1986) Survival in Down's syndrome. J Ment Defic Res 30:101–110
Giel R, Dijk S, van Weerden-Dijkstra JR (1978) Mortality in the long-stay population of all Dutch mental hospitals. Acta Psychiatr Scand 57:361–368
Gilmore AJJ (1975) Some characteristics of non-surviving subjects in a three-year longitudinal study of elderly people living at home. Geront Clin 17:72–79
Go RCP, Todorov AB, Elston RC, Constantinidis J (1978) The malignancy of dementias. Ann Neurol 3:559–561

Gopalaswamy AK, Morgan R (1985) Too many chronic mentally disabled patients are too fat. Acta Psychiatr Scand 72:254–258

Hagnell O, Lanke J, Rorsman B (1981) Suicide rates in the Lundby study: mental illness as a risk factor for suicide. Neuropsychobiology 7:248–253

Hall RCW, Popkin MK, Devaul RA, Faillace LA, Stickney SK (1978) Physical illness presenting as psychiatric disease. Arch Gen Psychiatry 35:1315–1320

Hall RCW, Gardner ER, Stickney SK, LeCann AF, Popkin MK (1980) Physical illness manifesting as psychiatric disease. II. Analysis of a State Hospital inpatient population. Arch Gen Psychiatry 37:989–995

Halldin J, Björk K, Lindeberg A (1985) Mortality in an urban population in central Sweden in relation to mental disorder and alcohol consumption. Acta Psychiatr Scand 72:374–381

Haugland G, Craig TJ, Goodman AB, Siegel C (1983) Mortality in the era of deinstitutionalization. Am J Psychiatry 140:848–852

Hawton K (1987) Assessment of suicide risk. Br J Psychiatry 150:145–153

Herrman HE, Baldwin JA, Christie D (1983) A record-linkage study of mortality and general hospital discharge in patients diagnosed as schizophrenic. Psychol Med 13:581–593

Hessö R (1977) Suicide in Norwegian, Finnish, and Swedish psychiatric hospitals. Arch Psychiatr Nervenkr 224:119–127

Heston LL (1981) Genetic studies of dementia: with emphasis on Parkinson's disease and Alzheimer's neuropathology. In: Mortimer JA, Schumann LM (eds) The epidemiology of dementia. Oxford University Press, New York, pp 101–114

Heston LL, Mastri AR, Anderson VE, White J (1981) Dementia of the Alzheimer type: clinical genetics, natural history and associated conditions. Arch Gen Psychiatry 38:1085–1090

Hsu LKG (1980) Outcome of anorexia nervosa. A review of the literature (1954 to 1978). Arch Gen Psychiatry 37:1041–1046

Innes G, Millar WM (1970) Mortality among psychiatric patients. Scott Med J 15:143–148

Jarvik LF, Ruth V, Matsuyama SS (1980) Organic brain syndrome and aging. Arch Gen Psychiatry 37:280–286

Kang J, Lemaire H-G, Unterbeck A, Salbaum JM, Masters CL, Multhaup G, Beyreuther K, Müller-Hill B (1987) The precursor of Alzheimer's disease amyloid A4 protein resembles a cell-surface receptor. Nature 325:733–736

Kaszniak AW, Fox J, Gandell DL, Garron DC, Huckman MS, Ramsey RG (1978) Predictors of mortality in presenile and senile dementia. Ann Neurol 3:246–252

Katona CLE, Lowe D, Jack RL (1983) Prediction of outcome in psychogeriatric patients. Acta Psychiatr Scand 67:297–306

Kay DWK, Bergmann K (1966) Physical disability and mental health in old age. A follow-up of a random sample of elderly people seen at home. J Psychosom Res 10:3–12

Kendler KS (1986) A twin study of mortality in schizophrenia and neurosis. Arch Gen Psychiatry 43:643–649

Kerr TA, Schapira K, Roth M (1969) The relationship between premature death and affective disorders. Br J Psychiatry 115:1277–1282

Koranyi EK (1980) Somatic illness in psychiatric patients. Psychosomatics 21:887–891

Kraft DP, Babigian HM (1976) Suicide by persons with and without psychiatric contacts. Arch Gen Psychiatry 33:209–215

Langley GE, Bayatti NN (1984) Suicides in Exe Vale Hospital 1972–1981. Br J Psychiatry 145:463–467

Larsson T, Sjögren T (1954) A methodological, psychiatric and statistical study of a large Swedish rural population. Acta Psychiatr Neurol Scand [Suppl] 89

Lipowski ZJ (1975) Psychiatry of somatic diseases: epidemiology pathogenesis, classification. Compr Psychiatry 16:105–124

Magnusson H, Helgason T (1981) Epidemiology of mental disorders in the aged on Iceland. In: Magnussen G, Nielsen J, Buch J (eds) Epidemiology and prevention of mental illness in old age. Nordisk Samråd for Aeldreaktivitet, Hellerup, pp 29–33

Malzberg B (1953) Further studies of mortality among patients with mental disease. Acta Med Scand 145 [Suppl]:215–230
Martin RL, Cloninger CR, Guze SB, Clayton PJ (1985 a) Mortality in a follow-up of 500 psychiatric outpatients. I Total mortality. Arch Gen Psychiatry 42:47–54
Martin RL, Cloninger CR, Guze SB, Clayton PJ (1985 b) Mortality in a follow-up of 500 psychiatric outpatients. II Cause-specific mortality. Arch Gen Psychiatry 42:58–66
Modestin J (1982) Suizid in der psychiatrischen Institution. Nervenarzt 53:254–261
Mölsä PK, Marttila RJ, Rinne UK (1986) Survival and cause of death in Alzheimer's disease and multi-infarct dementia. Acta Neurol Scand 74:103–107
Müller C (1981) Psychische Erkrankungen und ihr Verlauf sowie ihre Beeinflussung durch das Alter. Huber, Bern
Murphy JM, Monson RR, Olivier DC, Sobol AM, Leighton AH (1987) Affective disorders and mortality. A general population study. Arch Gen Psychiatry 44:473–480
Nakane Y, Ohta Y (1986) The example of linkage with a cancer register. In: ten Horn GHMM, Giel R, Gulbinat WH, Henderson JH (eds) Psychiatric case registers in public health. Elsevier, Amsterdam, pp 240–245
Nielsen J, Homma A, Biörn-Henriksen T (1977) Follow-up 15 years after a geronto-psychiatric prevalence study. Conditions concerning death, cause of death, and life expectancy in relation to psychiatric diagnosis. J Gerontol 32:554–561
Ödegård Ö (1936) Mortality in Norwegian mental hospitals from 1916 to 1933. Acta Psychiatr Scand 11:323–356
Ödegård Ö (1951) Mortality in Norwegian mental hospitals 1926–1941. Acta Genet (Basel) 2:141–173
Ödegård Ö (1952) The excess mortality of the insane. Acta Psychiatr Neurol Scand 27:353–367
Ödegård Ö (1967) Mortality in Norwegian psychiatric hospitals 1950–1962. Acta Genet (Basel) 17:137–153
Perris C, Beskow J, Jacobsson L (1980) Some remarks on the incidence of successful suicide in psychiatric cases. Soc Psychiatry 15:161–166
Persson G (1981) Five-year mortality in a 70-year-old urban population in relation to psychiatric diagnosis, personality, sexuality and early parental death. Acta Psychiatr Scand 64:244–253
Ribourdouille M, Corten P (1986) Mortalité chez des patients fréquentant un secteur psychiatrique. Acta Psychiatr Belg 86:514–525
Rorsman B (1974) Mortality among psychiatric patients. Acta Psychiatr Scand 50:354–375
Rorsman B, Hagnell O, Lanke J (1982) Mortality in the Lundby study. Natural death in different forms of mental disorder in a total population investigated during a 25-year period. Neuropsychobiology 8:188–197
Rorsman B, Hagnell O, Lanke J (1983) Mortality and psychiatric specialist care in the Lundby study. Age-standardized death rates in different forms of psychiatric services in a total population investigated during a 25-year period. Neuropsychobiology 9:2–8
Rorsman B, Hagnell O, Lanke J (1985) Prevalence of age psychosis and mortality among age psychotics in the Lundby study. Change over time during a 25-year observation period. Neuropsychobiology 13:167–172
Roth M (1955) The natural history of mental disorder in old age. J Ment Sci 101:281–301
Saugstad LF, Ödegård Ö (1979) Mortality in psychiatric hospitals in Norway 1950–74. Acta Psychiatr Scand 59:431–447
Saugstad L, Ödegård Ö (1985) Recent rise in supposedly stress dependent causes of death in psychiatric hospitals in Norway indicating increased "stress" in hospitals? Acta Psychiatr Scand 71:402–409
Schmidt W, de Lint J (1969) Mortality experiences of male and female alcoholic patients. J Stud Alcohol 30:112–118
Schmidtke A, Häfner H (1985) Do cohort effects influence suicide rates? Arch Gen Psychiatry 42:926–927
Schwalb H, Eckmann F, Brüninghaus H (1981) Psychopharmaka und kardiale Risikofaktoren. Nervenarzt 52:549–553

Shaw S, Sims A (1984) A survey of unexpected deaths among psychiatric in-patients and ex-patients. Br J Psychiatry 146:473–476
Similae S, von Wendt L, Rantakallio P (1986) Mortality of mentally retarded children to 17 years of age assessed in a prospective one-year birth cohort. J Ment Defic Res 30:401–405
Sims A (1978) Hypotheses linking neuroses with premature mortality. Psychol Med 8:255–263
Sims A (1984) Neuroses and mortality: investigating an association. J Psychosom Res 28:353–362
Sims A, Prior P (1978) The pattern of mortality in severe neuroses. Br J Psychiatry 133:299–305
Singer E, Garfinkel R, Cohen MS, Srole L (1976) Mortality and mental health: evidence from the Midtown Manhattan restudy. Soc Sci Med 10:517–525
Steinhausen H-C, Glanville K (1983) Follow-up studies of anorexia nervosa: a review of research findings. Editorial. Psychol Med 13:239–249
Tait D (1983) Mortality and dementia among ageing defectives. J Ment Defic Res 27:133–142
Taylor JR, Combs-Orme T, Taylor DA (1983) Alcohol and mortality. Diagnostic considerations. J Stud Alcohol 44:17–25
Tokuhata GK, Stehman VA (1958) Mortality in state mental hospitals of Michigan, 1950–54. Public Health Rep 73:750–761
Tsuang MT (1978) Suicide in schizophrenics, maniacs, depressives, and surgical controls. A comparison with general population suicide mortality. Arch Gen Psychiatry 35:153–155
Tsuang MT, Simpson JC (1985) Mortality studies in psychiatry. Should they stop or proceed? Arch Gen Psychiatry 42:98–103
Tsuang MT, Woolson RF, Fleming JA (1980) Premature deaths in schizophrenia and affective disorders. An analysis of survival curves and variables affecting the shortened survival. Arch Gen Psychiatry 37:979–983
Tsuang MT, Perkins KP, Simpson JC (1983) Physical diseases in schizophrenia and affective disorders. J Clin Psychiatry 44:42–46
Vitaliano PP, Peck A, Johnson DA, Prinz PN, Eisdorfer C (1981) Dementia and other competing risks for mortality in the institutionalized aged. J Am Geriatr Soc 29:513–519
Wood JB, Evenson RC, Cho DW, Hagan BJ (1985) Mortality variations among public mental health patients. Acta Psychiatr Scand 72:218–229
World Health Organization (1986) Summary report. Working group on preventive practices in suicide and attempted suicide. WHO, Copenhagen (ICP/PSF 017 (S), 6526 V)

Discussion in Connection with Häfner and Bickel's Paper: Physical Mortality and Morbidity in Psychiatric Patients

B. RORSMAN

One of the most solid facts available in psychiatry is the repeatedly confirmed finding that there is an excess mortality among both previous and current psychiatric patients. Even this basic and concrete fact is, however, not quite clear, but remains ambiguous. Death by suicide or accident can be considered as a fairly direct consequence of a mental disorder, but the association between a mental disorder and death from natural causes is more complex and puzzling.

When it comes to samples of psychiatric patients, it can be argued that the excess physical mortality might not be associated with the mental disorder per se but may, totally or partly, be explained by the mere fact that the probands in question are psychiatric patients. There are many selective factors that might play a role in this respect. Emotionally disturbed people may seek advice concerning their physical illness more easily than those who are emotionally stable, while persons with concurrent somatic and psychiatric symptoms are probably more prone to be referred for psychiatric care. Within all types of psychiatric services, there is thus a selection of physically vulnerable persons, with a high potential risk of physical illness and thus premature death.

The problem concerning physical mortality and the biases associated with the status of being a psychiatric patient are, in a sense, analogous to the main problem in epidemiological research. Instead of relying on patient samples, epidemiologists are interested in treated as well as untreated cases, and try to calculate the "true" incidence and prevalence of mental disorder in the community. Some recent epidemiological studies have in fact tried to determine the relationship between mental health and excess mortality in general population samples.

Two well-known longitudinal studies in the United States and Canada – the Midtown Manhattan Restudy and the Stirling County Study – have recently reported the results of a follow-up investigation of mortality. Both studies used structured interviews for identifying psychiatric illness, but the results arrived at were contradictory.

The Midtown Manhattan Restudy was published by Singer et al. in 1976. Persons rated for mental health in 1954 were studied in relation to mortality

Department of Psychiatry and Neurochemistry, University of Lund, Box 638, S-22006 Lund

Interaction Between Mental and Physical Illness
Edited by R. Öhman et al.

during the next 20 years. In addition to age and sex, many variables were controlled, such as marital and economic status, education, and drinking habits. The investigators concluded that:

> The present study makes clear that the associations previously reported between treated mental illness and premature or excess mortality do not prevail in the general population, when variables related both to mental illness and to mortality are controlled ... The most likely explanation is that mental illness is related to excess mortality only in its more severe manifestations, or only when it is accompanied by behavior injurious to health – e.g. alcohol abuse.

It should be added that the most powerful predictor of mortality among the variables examined was a markedly reduced probability of dying among those who in 1954 considered themselves to be in "excellent" health.

The mortality experience of the Stirling County population has been studied by Murphy et al. (1987), and an increased death risk was in fact found from natural as well as unnatural causes.

The Stirling County Study is a 16-year prospective examination of a general population sample, followed-up during the period 1952 to 1968: those who had reported a depression with or without anxiety at the baseline in 1952 experienced about one and a half times the number of deaths expected from a large reference population. Sex, age, and self-reported physical health at the baseline were controlled for. An increased total death risk was found to be significantly associated with affective but not physical disorders, and with depression but not generalized anxiety. The relationship between depression and death was significantly more pronounced in men: among depressed men, the risk of dying of a cardiovascular disorder was twice that expected. Comparing their findings with the standardized total mortality ratios for primary affective disorder in American psychiatric patient samples, such as those recently published from Iowa and St. Louis, the authors comment that "on the whole, our findings suggest that disorders identified in a community survey may carry a risk that is similar to that observed among psychiatric patients."

In a mortality study from the Lundby Study (Rorsman et al. 1983), we have chosen to investigate treated and untreated mentally ill probands separately.

The Lundby Study is a 25-year follow-up investigation of a normal Swedish population of 3563 persons. The case ascertainment was carried out through clinical interviews performed by psychiatrists in 1947, 1957, and 1972. The total cohort was divided into three subgroups: (a) psychiatric patients, i.e., persons with a background of psychiatric care during the observation period (all types of facilities were included, as well as contact with psychiatrists in private practice); (b) mentally ill psychiatric nonpatients, i.e., persons meeting the Lundby criteria for "caseness," but who had not received any psychiatric treatment or attention (persons with alcoholism, a personality disorder, or mental retardation were not counted as "cases"); (c) the rest, i.e., "healthy" in the restricted sense that they had neither been "cases" nor "patients" during the observation period. The findings are given in Table 1. In both sexes, psychiatric patients show a significantly increased natural death risk. Mentally ill men who have not been psychiatric patients run a relative risk that is even more

Table 1. Natural death in the Lundby cohort followed during 25 and 15 years, respectively, and in three subgroups of the cohort

	Age-standardized natural death rate/ 100000 person-years	Natural death rate relative to rate in total cohort
Men		
Psychiatric patient	1065	1.5*
Psychiatric nonpatient	1215	1.7***
"Healthy"	553	0.76***
Total Lundby male cohort	731	
Women		
Psychiatric patient	1124	1.5*
Psychiatric nonpatient	890	1.2
"Healthy"	631	0.84***
Total Lundby female cohort	751	

Psychiatric patients, persons with a background of psychiatric care (all types of services); mentally ill psychiatric nonpatients, persons meeting the Lundby criteria for "caseness" without a background of psychiatric care; "Healthy," persons not meeting the Lundby criteria for "caseness" and without a background of psychiatric care
* $P<0.05$; *** $P<0.001$

marked than the risk run by male psychiatric patients, while untreated mentally ill women show a risk that only slightly exceeds the one expected. In the "healthy" group, the risk of dying was significantly decreased.

The findings from Lundby are very similar to those from Stirling County. These general population studies both indicate that, at least in men, treated as well as untreated mental disorder strongly affects the probability of dying of natural causes. In agreement with the Midtown Manhattan Restudy, we found that for both the sexes, mental health is a very powerful protective predictive factor.

The three studies mentioned cover mainly the 1950s, 1960s, and early 1970s, after which time traditional psychiatry has undergone profound changes. Psychiatric outpatient treatment is more easily available for everybody, and in addition, doctors in primary care are nowadays probably more aware of psychiatric problems and more prone to diagnose and treat them, especially depressions, than they were before. Recent mortality studies based on findings in psychiatric patients indicate that the mortality risk in this group may be declining. It must be hoped that in the future, more of the mentally disturbed persons in the general population will receive effective psychiatric as well as medical help.

The presentation by Häfner and Bickel underlines the fact that psychiatry is a branch of medicine; the clinical psychiatrist has a great responsibility in the search for prophylactic measures, and psychiatrists will have to cooperate more than before with their medical colleagues. Contributions from basic biology and from all scientific fields that deal with human behavior will also be required.

It is a difficult task to choose the most needed areas of future research in this very heterogeneous field. I agree that prospective studies are very important, and in relation to the problem of psychiatric mortality, we need more prospective studies, focused on specific diagnostic groups or on well-described syndromes and diagnosis-specific causes of death. Close cooperation between psychiatrists, pathologists, and other professionals will be necessary in order to follow large samples of carefully studied subgroups of psychiatric disorder, and to evaluate and assess causes of death. In addition, precipitating as well as protecting environmental and psychological factors ought to be analysed. Such studies are time-consuming and costly but may, in the long run, give fruitful results.

References

Murphy JM, Monson RR, Olivier DC, Sobol AM, Leighton AH (1987) Affective disorders and mortality. A general population study. Arch Gen Psychiatry 44:473–480

Rorsman B, Hagnell O, Lanke J (1983) Mortality and hidden mental disorder in the Lundby study. Age-standardized death rates among mentally ill "non-patients" in a total population observed during a 25-year period. Neuropsychobiology 10:83–89

Singer E, Garfinkel R, Cohen SM, Srole L (1976) Mortality and mental health: evidence from the Midtown Manhatten restudy. Soc Sci Med 10:517–525

Hypothesis Concerning "Natural" Mortality in Psychiatry

PH. CORTEN and M. RIBOURDOUILLE

The high mortality rate amongst psychiatric patients has been a well-known phenomenon for a long time (Esquirol 1838; Griesinger 1865; Cullere 1890; von Kraft-Ebing 1897). In 1838, Esquirol had already underlined the problem at the Bicêtre Hospital between 1784–1794 (Esquirol 1838), while the first paper on the subject using statistical methods dates from 1841 (Farr 1841). The first question is whether or not the phenomenon of high mortality still exists today: Craig and Lin (1981) have described an excess death rate in a psychiatric population in New York both before and after the introduction of psychotropic drugs.

Secondly, the importance of the problem in terms of public health needs to be known. The phenomenon seems to be of greater importance than previously suspected. Indeed, the risk of death during the year following the first psychiatric episode (139 per thousand, cf Craig 1981) may be similar to the risk of death 24 h to 1 year after a heart attack (142 per thousand computed from WHO 1979). Hagnell (1966) found that 4 out of 10 men and 7 out of 10 women will have at least one psychiatric episode between the age of 10 and 60 years; this indicates the size of the population at risk.

Since death by suicide is well known in psychiatric patients, the third question is whether or not this excess mortality rate is limited to suicide. This does not seem likely as, even if one excludes suicides and accidents, the risk remains two to five times greater than normal. In addition, Teft (1977), in an epidemiological study in New York between 1960 and 1970, provided evidence that the rate for death by suicide within a psychiatric population (excluding those who had attempted suicide previously) is very near normal.

The last question is whether this high mortality rate is not simply due to ageing of the hospitalized population. It is not: (a) because the same phenomenon is observed amongst patients who are not hospitalized (Amdur and Souchek 1981; Babigian and Odoroff 1969; Koranyi 1977; Raymond et al. 1981; Ribourdouille and Corten 1986; Rorsman 1974; Weiner and Warvit 1977), and (b) because this high death rate is not as pronounced among older patients (Ödegård 1967).

École de Santé Publique, U. L. B., 808 Route de Lennik, B-1070 Bruxelles

Interaction Between Mental and Physical Illness
Edited by R. Öhman et al.

Aims

The aim of our study was to analyse the phenomenon of supposedly natural excess mortality rates. To do this we chose to review the international literature on this subject, most of which is essentially descriptive. Our aim here was to go beyond the level of descriptive statistics, in order to extract from the texts the main substance that would enable us to put forward some hypotheses.

Therefore, we analyzed these articles, keeping in mind three essential questions:

1. What are the persistent phenomena?
2. What changes are there?
3. What are the risk factors?

Methodological Problems

A major methodological problem encountered in all studies based on bibliographical review here is the heterogeneity of the data to be evaluated. It is not only the methods and evaluation of results that differ, but concepts may also differ considerably from one study to another. There is no universal definition of what constitutes a mentally ill person. Notions of in- and outpatients are largely attributable to the health care system in use in the region studied, and even if we compare identical types of services, they may differ from one country to another, or even within the same country.

Therefore, the only role of a bibliographical comparison can be to make new suppositions and guide research in new directions.

Data

Persistence of the Phenomenon of a High Mortality Rate

As mentioned above, this phenomenon has been observed over a long period of time (Esquirol 1838; Griesinger 1865; Shepherd 1957; Ekblom and Frisk 1960; Niswander et al. 1963; Hoenig and Hamilton 1966; Savnino and Brody 1966; Ödegård 1967; Tsuang and Woolson 1977; Saugstad and Ödegård 1979; Craig and Lin 1981; Ryan 1982). As Table 1 shows, the phenomenon has also been observed throughout the world, though with certain important variations in the death rate, probably due to the date of the study, but also to the different methodologies used. The phenomenon seems to be equally observable in urban and rural settings (Ekblom and Frisk 1960; Westermeyer 1978). However, no reports of comparable studies are available from developing countries. No ethnic group seems to escape this phenomenon (Babigian and Odoroff 1969; Weiner and Warvit 1977; Gottschalk et al. 1979; Amdur and Souchek 1981).

Table 1. Mortality in psychiatry, a universal phenomenon

Year	Length of the follow-up	Country	Author	Sample	Deaths	Excess mortality	
						Men	Women
1841		United Kingdom	Farr (1841)			6.5	
1916–1941	1 to 25 years	Norway	Ödegård (1951)	21 522 inp	3 367	4.7	5.5
1950–1954	4 years	Michigan, USA	Tokuhata and Stehman (1958)			3.4	3.2
1950–1962	13 years	Norway	Ödegård (1967)	8 650 per year	4 251	2.9	3.2
1959–1968	10 years	Birmingham, UK	Sims (1973)	1 482 inp	139	1.7	
1960–1966	7 years	New York, USA	Babigian and Odoroff (1969)	39 475 inp-out	3 809	2.5	2.9
1962–1968	6 years	Sweden	Rorsman (1974)	757 inp	56	1.9	1.6
			Rorsman et al. (1982)	2 866 out	204	1.8	1.4
1962–1972	10 years	Hawaii, USA	Weiner and Warvit (1977)	1 689 inp-out	219	1.9	
1963–1974	11 years	Norway	Saugstad and Ödegård (1979)		6 257	3.6	2.5
1964–1974	10 years	Genèva, Switz.	Raymond et al. (1981)	1 466 out	238	1.8	2.0
1968–1970	3 years	Tokyo, Japan	Shinozaki (1976)	10 199 inp	1 143	6.8	7.5
1969–1971	min 4 years	Holland, Neth.	Giel et al. (1978)	17 211 inp	1 506	1.68	1.85
1969–1977	8 years	New York, USA	Craig and Lin (1980)		2 054	2.6	3.3
1972–1975	3 years	Ottawa, Canada	Koranyi (1979)	2 070 out	28	2.0	
1972–1978	27 to 72 months	Chicago, USA	Amdur and Souchek (1981)	820 out	58	3.4	
1973–1983	10 years	Brussels, Belgium	Ribourdouille and Corten (1986)	308 out	15	5.05	5.63

inp, inpatients; out, outpatients

As far as sex is concerned, some studies have found a significantly higher rate of mortality among men (Singer et al. 1976; Craig 1981), sometimes as much as three times than among women (Amdur and Souchek 1981), while others have found the opposite to be the case (Alstrom 1942; Ödegård 1967; Ciompi and Medvecka 1976) (Table 1).

Early studies hypothesized that the high rate of death was due to conditions of institutionalization, but it was shown that similar findings were also observed among outpatients (Babigian and Odoroff 1969; Rorsman 1974; Koranyi 1977; Weiner and Warvit 1977; Amdur and Souchek 1981; Raymond et al. 1981; Ribourdouille and Corten 1986; Corten et al. 1986). However, these studies do not indicate whether or not the severity of the out-patients' illness was comparable with that of the hospitalized patients. Moreover, it appears from several epidemiological studies that at least two groups of individuals coexist within the population: a first group using hospital facilities and a second preferring to attend as outpatients. These two groups rarely overlap (Ferrero et al. 1986; Lacrosse et al. 1984; Hermann 1986). The problem becomes all the more complex if we want to compare the situations in different countries which have health systems that are not comparable.

Generally, psychoorganic syndromes are illnesses that have a very high risk of mortality (standard mortality ratios of up to 25; Wood et al. 1985). Nevertheless, even those psychiatric illnesses without an organic substrate have an excess mortality rate. The studies are unanimous with regard to this increased mortality (Ödegård 1952; Malzberg 1953; Babigian and Odoroff 1969; Innes and Millar 1970; Gross 1971; Sims 1973; Rorsman 1974; Ciompi and Medvecka 1976; Wood et al. 1985), but are not in accord about the relative risks of different psychiatric illnesses.

Elevated Incidence During the First Year of Psychiatric Illness

The large number of deaths occurring during the first year of illness (Table 2) is a characteristic which exists in all known times and places. Ödegård (1951), Malzberg (1953), Hoenig and Hamilton (1966), Savino and Brody (1966), Innes and Millar (1970), Tarjan (in Watkins et al. 1972), Rorsman (1974) and Craig and Lin (1981) confirm this also in relation to type of treatment (in- or outpatient). Savino and Brody (1966), who studied the number of deaths in Californian hospitals during the past 100 years, also have concluded that the first year was always the most critical. In contrast to these findings, Sims (1984) showed that in a group of neurotic patients, the mortality rate, excluding suicide and accidental death, started at a level similar to that of the normal population and gradually increased, stabilizing during the fourth year. In addition to the specific population studied (patients with neurosis) Sims eliminated from the follow-up those who, at the beginning of the study, had some type of physical problem. Therefore, his sample was not representative of most psychiatric populations.

Table 2. Excess mortality during the first year

Author	Sex	1st year	2nd year	Population reference
Esquirol (1838)		48.35%		Deaths
Ödegård (1951)	M	10.0[a]	5.6[a]	
	F	10.4[a]	6.0[a]	
Sheperd (1957)		59.0%		Deaths
		84.3%		Deaths
Malzberg (1953)	M	34.53%	10.16%	Deaths
	F	28.41%	9.98%	Deaths
Hoenig and Hamilton (1966)		44.5%		Deaths
Innes and Millar (1970)	M	43.8%	17.6%	Deaths
	F	39.3%	13.6%	Deaths
Craig and Lin (1981)		13.8%	3.8%	Population
Ribourdouille and Corten (1986)		53.3%	13.3%	Deaths

[a] Relative risk

Table 3. Standard mortality ratio (SMR) by age group (computed from Ödegård 1967)

Age group (years)	Women	Men
20–29	21.20	4.77
30–39	11.89	4.25
40–49	7.00	3.61
50–59	5.33	2.76
60–69	4.23	3.05
70–79	2.27	2.96

Risk Among Young Adults

The mortality rate is not the same for all age groups (Table 3). The relative excess risk of death seems to decrease with age, with the greatest risk being for those between the ages of 20 and 29, followed by those between 30 and 39. This was confirmed by Ödegård (1967), Malzberg (1953), Innes and Millar (1970), Rorsman (1974) and Craig (1981).

Sudden and Unexpected Death

While mortality has been observed statistically in psychiatric populations, including all diagnoses, it has not been the subject of many clinical studies. The

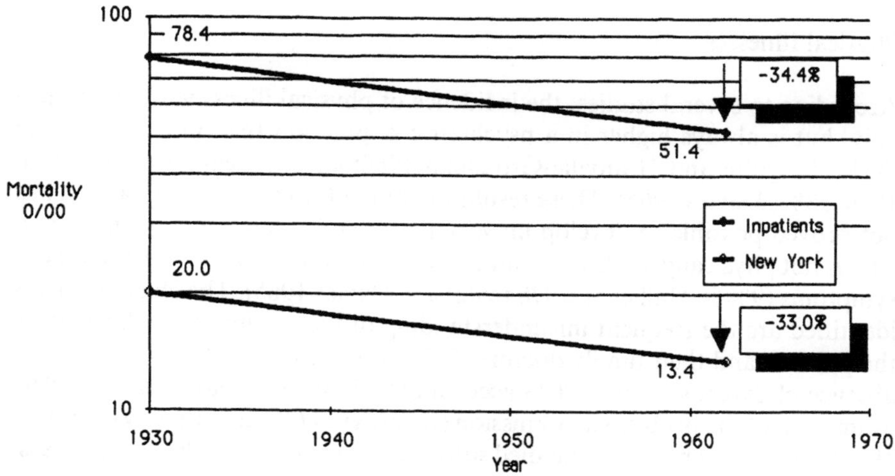

Fig. 1. Standardized mortality rate (New York, Kramer)

sudden aspect of these deaths has been emphasized since Esquirol (1838) and Griesinger (1865). Some studies provide evidence for the existence of sudden death (Hussar 1962; Hollister and Kosek 1965; Richardson et al. 1966; Ellman 1982), while there are also deaths from known causes, where the illness would not otherwise have been expected to produce that result.

What Changes Have Occurred?

Although the high mortality rate in psychiatric patients has always existed, it is also true that there has been a marked decrease since 1950, which may be due to better living conditions and medical progress. If the pattern of death rates of hospitalized psychiatric patients is compared with that of the population of New York between 1930 and 1962 (Fig. 1), it can be seen that both have decreased in the same proportions (34%, Kramer 1970). At the same time, there have been profound changes since 1950 in the psychiatric population. The age of hospitalized patients has increased, as has the proportion of organic and nonpsychotic cases. Over the years, many other factors have also been modified, such as lifestyle, eating habits, effects of pollution, etc.

It must be emphasized that while populations observed during different epochs are being analysed here, we are not referring to the same population. No study has standardized the death rate by diagnosis made during each epoch.

What Are the Risk Factors?

Certain risk factors are recognized unanimously, such as alcohol and drug-related problems and concomitant physical illnesses. Others, such as sociological variables, are considered risk factors only in some studies and not in others.

Physical Illnesses

According to several studies, the incidence of physical illness varies considerably, but is always higher in a psychiatric population than in a normal one (33%, Maguire and Granville-Grossman 1968; 42%, Hoenig and Hamilton 1966; 58%, Davies 1965). These results are difficult to compare, because it has not proved possible to develop universal criteria for determining who is and who is not physically ill. Physical illnesses are often the cause of the psychiatric symptoms (9% in Hall et al. 1978 to 42% in Davies 1965). The chief problems identified are the frequent misunderstanding of the nature of the illnesses by the patients and their family doctors (50% according to Hall et al. 1978); the absence of diagnosis (up to 80% according to Johnson 1968); and the underestimation of the problem at admission (Koranyi 1977). In one study (Koranyi 1977), 80% of the patients who died suffered from associated physical diseases, of which one-third were undiagnosed even at autopsy. The most frequently associated physical diseases cited are cardiovascular and endocrine disorders (such as diabetes, Hall et al. 1978; Koranyi 1979) and organic brain syndromes (Herridge 1960).

Obesity and Hypertension

Singer et al. (1976) has shown that after age, educational level, and sex, obesity and hypertension are the factors most predictive of mortality.

Alcohol and Drug-Related Problems

The role of the consequences of addiction as a risk factor no longer needs to be demonstrated, whether it is associated with drugs or, more often, alcohol. In fact, it further multiplies by two (Babigian and Odoroff 1969) or three (Amdur and Souchek 1981) the risk of death for a psychiatric patient, whereas that risk is already at least double that of a subject from the general population.

Sociological Variables

As far as marital status is concerned, the fact of living alone and isolated, without family or friends, and without a supporting social structure, is a risk factor (Amdur and Souchek 1981). This characteristic does not seem to be limited to mental illnesses, as Koskenvuo et al. (1979) have found a higher mortality rate for all causes for divorced men and women in the general population in Finland, in comparison with other marital status. Concerning socioeconomic status, it is notable that coming from a lower social class when the first symptoms appear seems to be a risk factor (Sims 1973; Singer et al. 1976; Leclerc et al. 1979). Sims (1979) and Rorsman (1974) have shown the impact of financial problems and unemployment among patients who had died.

Hypothesis

Tested Hypothesis

Toxicity of Psychotropic Medication

Both Table 1 and Fig. 1 demonstrate that while psychotropic medication did not really lower the death rate, it did not aggravate the problem either (Zlotlow and Paganini 1958; Hussar 1962; Turunen and Salminen 1968; Babigian and Odoroff 1969; Glen et al. 1979; Craig and Lin 1980, 1981). In fact, the stability of the number of deaths seems to support the nontoxicity, in the long term, of the new medication (Brill and Patton 1962; Glen et al. 1979).

Some authors have mentioned sudden death associated with the taking of phenothiazines (Hussar 1962; Hollister and Kosek 1965; Richardson et al. 1966; Ellman 1982), but studies that compared this phenomenon with a control group or with the general population have been unable to show a correlation. Avery and Winokur (1976) have shown a reduced risk from death by natural causes or by suicide in a population of depressive patients correctly treated with electroconvulsive therapy and/or tricyclics.

Life Habits

Psychiatric populations consume more tobacco and alcohol than the general population, and these risk factors decrease their life expectancy. Cochet and Raymond (1985), however, have found that in a psychiatric population (alcoholics excluded), there was no higher mortality rate due to cirrhosis or bronchial cancer, which seemed to invalidate this hypothesis. Singer et al. (1976) also have shown that cigarette smoking does not seem to be a risk factor among the mentally ill, though this is disputed by Salmon and Sims (1981).

Untested Hypothesis

An Eventual Correlation Between the Intensity of the Last Event Experienced and Death

It would seem that these two findings are not related from the point of view of intensity, but rather that death is due to a "last straw" phenomenon. Confronted with some final event, the person can no longer handle the situation, which would result in the early development of a physical disease, that was inevitable in any case (Sims and Prior 1978). The difficulty of this approach, however, is to demonstrate its relevance.

Perception of Physical Symptoms

The insensitivity of schizophrenics to pain and cold has been known for some time (Ey et al. 1970). It might be concluded from this that this lack of perception of physical problems would be the cause of the failure of early diagnosis of a physical illness by the doctor and of its inescapable conclusion. However, contrary to information sometimes expressed, spontaneous use of medical services by the mentally ill is known to be equal to if not superior to that of the nonpsychiatric population. On the other hand, psychotherapy tends to result in a decreased consumption of these services (Follet and Cummings 1967; Goldberg and Blackwell 1970; Duehrssen and Jorswieck 1975; Jameson et al. 1978; Cronholm and Daly 1983).

Explanatory Theories

Sims (1985) has reviewed several psychosomatic theories dealing with the phenomenon of natural mortality as giving up – rejected, alexithymia, Type A pattern of behavior, etc. To our knowledge, no study has attempted to test these various theories. There is nothing to exclude the possibility that some mental diseases may be lethal in themselves. In fact the causes of mortality among psychiatric patients do not necessarily correspond to the causes of death in the general population (Hussar 1962; Shinozaki 1976).

Perspectives

For reasons of clarity and because they are closely related, we have divided these hypotheses along two axes; the psychosocial and the psychobiological.

Psychosocial Axis

Decrease in the Perception of Somatic Symptoms by Some of the Mentally Ill

Since the requirements for medical care of psychiatric patients are not less than those of the general population, we must determine whether or not these patients describe their symptoms adequately.

Disregard by Doctors of the Somatic Complaints of the Mentally Ill

The mentally ill patient, due to his difficulties in relationships and possible disturbances in his speech, is not an easy subject for investigation and medical history. This situation often invites rejection and disregard of complaints. For instance, 20% of the patients who come to the casualty ward of a general hospital with psychosomatic complaints do not undergo a physical examination (Corten and Pelc 1984).

Also, somatic symptoms may be profoundly altered, perhaps even completely absent, as a result of drug treatment or due to psychiatric illnesses (afebrile pneumonia due to the hypothermic effect of the neuroleptics, diabetic polydipsia hidden by the anticholinergic effect of certain medications, peritonitis with a supple abdomen, etc.).

Role of Friends and Family

In the case of psychiatric patients, do friends and family play an alerting role regarding the disturbing symptoms which often, as opposed to the case with nonpsychiatric patients, bring them to the doctor? Patients who come to the casualty ward of a general hospital, for example, psychiatric emergencies are only accompanied by a family member in 9% of cases (Corten et al. 1981).

Difficulty of Changing Behavior

The diagnosis of a chronic physical illness often requires modification of lifestyle. The obese must become more active and eat less; the hypertensive patient must decrease salt intake and change the rhythm of his life. One may well ask if such changes in lifestyle are possible for those people undergoing a psychological crisis or who are chronically disturbed.

Biological Axis

Throughout this review we have been able to show how the increased number of deaths have had an abnormal character (young adult populations, sudden death, abnormally catastrophic course), but we have not been able to show the specific cause of death. Future research must be orientated towards homeostatic mechanisms, such as those described in models like the theory of stress by Selye (1974) or the general system approach of von Bertalanffy (1968).

As far as we can tell, some approaches are favored by the scientific world, and could enable us to make progress. These include, for instance, those studies dealing with disruptions of the hypothalamic-hypophyseal axes, but also research dealing with immunity collapse, and genetic studies.

Conclusions

Several interesting points and questions emanating from the three questions with which we started can be identified.

Persistence of the Phenomenon

The natural high mortality rate has always existed and is still observed now in every country, ethnic group, sex, age, or place of treatment. The psychoorganic syndromes appear to differ clearly from other mental illnesses with a very high mortality rate. Furthermore, two other findings merit a more detailed examination: the vulnerability of the young adult, and the unexpected aspect of death associated with the phenomenon. Finally, two observations seem, as yet, to be insufficiently studied: the comparison of in- and outpatients and the higher incidence of natural mortality during the first year of psychiatric illness.

Changes

If the excess mortality seems less important at the present time, the decrease is nonetheless closely proportional to that of the general population. It would therefore be of great interest to study the mortality differentials over a period of time, standardizing not only for age and sex, but also for diagnosis.

Risk Factors

Some sociological factors, observed elsewhere in nonpsychiatric populations, are also found here, the greater vulnerability of isolated people and the impact of socioeconomic factors, for example. Some physical factors are also encountered, such as obesity and arterial hypertension. Alcohol and drugs are also well known as aggravating factors. Lastly, it appears that the percentage of underestimated or undiagnosed physical illnesses is, even in the most optimistic studies, particularly elevated. A number of hypotheses can be raised here regarding the patient's own perception of somatic troubles, the doctor's underestimation of somatic complaints of a mentally ill patient, the alertness of those around the patient, and the possibility of modifying the psychiatric patient's life habits.

As for hypotheses, to our knowledge, only one seems to have been sufficiently tested, and it tends to disallow the toxicity of medication as a cause.

Hypotheses have been developed regarding the role of arteriosclerosis, life habits, and life events; all seem to show correlations that will need to be verified and studied. It seems surprising to note, for example, that even though psychiatric patients consume more tobacco than the general population, a high death rate from bronchial cancer is not observed.

The natural mortality rate in psychiatry does not seem to be associated with specific pathologies; rather, we tend to support the hypothesis of the heightened vulnerability of mentally ill patients. However, the probable interaction between mental illness and concomitant physical illness – declared or not – must be remembered. Thus, it would be of great interest to explore this hypothesis in greater depth from the systemic point of view.

It seems clear that, despite the quality of somatic care presently provided to the mentally ill, the natural death rate remains of great concern in terms of public health, being almost similar to that of heart attacks. Contrary to the current practice of psychiatric services, it seems imperative that psychiatric patients should have the benefit of a meticulous somatic follow-up during the first years of illness, whether they are hospitalized or not.

References

Alstrom CH (1942) Mortality in mental hospitals with special regard to tuberculosis. Acta Psychiatr Neurol Scand 17 [Suppl 24]:1–85

Amdur MA, Souchek J (1981) Death in aftercare. Compr Psychiatry 22(6):619–626

Avery D, Winokur G (1976) Mortality in depressed patients treated with electroconvulsive therapy and antidepressants. Arch Gen Psychiatry 33:1029–1037

Babigian HM, Odoroff CL (1969) The mortality experience of a population with psychiatric illness. Am J Psychiatry 126(4):470–480

Brill H, Patton RE (1962) Clinical-statistical analysis of population changes in New York State mental hospitals since introduction of psychotropic drugs. Am J Psychiatry 119:20–35

Ciompi L, Medvecka J (1976) Etude comparative de la mortalité à long terme des les maladies mentales. Arch Suisses Neurol Neurochir Psychiatr 118(1):111–135

Cochet B, Raymond L (1985) Mortalité en psychiatrie ambulatoire institutionnelle. Abstracts of the IIIrd international congress of the International Federation of Psychiatric Epidemiology, Brussels, p 82

Corten PhF, Pelc I (1984) Profil d'urgences psychiatriques à la garde d'hopitaux généraux. Acta Psychiatr Belg 84:483–499

Corten PhF, Pelc I, Vermeylen J (1981) Les urgences psy. In: Cahiers de psychologie médicale vol 1. Université Libre de Bruxelles, pp 1–75

Corten PhF, Hoyois P, Samoilovich F (1986) Evaluation du devenir des jeunes patients ayant été pris en charge par des structures intermédiaires. Acta Psychiatr Belg 86:394–401

Craig TJ, Lin SP (1980) Medication use and deaths attributed to asphyxia among psychiatric patients. Am J Psychiatry 137:1366–1373

Craig TJ, Lin SP (1981) Mortality among psychiatric inpatients. Age-adjusted comparison of populations before and after the psychotropic era. Arch Gen Psychiatry 38:935–938

Cronholm B, Daly RJ (1983) Evaluation of Psychiatric treatment. In: Helgasson T (ed) Methodology of evaluation of psychiatric treatment. Cambridge University Press, Cambridge, pp 3–32

Cullerre A (1890) Marche et terminaisons de la folie. Article III: complications. In: Traité pratique des maladies mentales. Baillière Paris, pp 90–95

Davies DW (1965) Physical illness in psychiatric out-patients. Br J Psychiatry 111:27–33

Duehrssen A, Jorswieck E (1975) An empirical-statistical investigation into the efficacity of psychoanalytic treatment. Nervenarzt 36:166–169

Ekblom B, Frisk M (1960) On changes in the death-risk in mental hospitals in Finland during the years 1920–1955. Acta Psychiatr Neurol Scand 36(2):300–324
Ellman JP (1982) Sudden death. Can J Psychiatry 27(4):331–333
Esquirol E (1838) II. Mémoires statistiques et hygiénique sur la folie (tome second)-XVII. Mémoire historique et statistique sur la Maison Royale de Charenton. In: Des maladies mentales. Tircher, Bruxelles, pp 284–291
Ey H, Bernard P, Bisset CH (1970) Manuel de psychiatrie. Masson, Paris
Farr W (1841) Report upon the mortality of lunatics. Journal of the Statistical Society 4(1):17–33
Ferrero F, Hermann P, Tricot L (1986) Analyse des trajectoires de soins d'une cohorte de 280 patients dépressifs. Acta Psychiatr Belg 86:381–387
Follet EW, Cummings NA (1967) Psychiatric services and medical utilization in a prepaid health plan setting. Med Care 5:25
Giel R, Dijk S, van Weerden D (1978) Mortality in the long-stay population of all Dutch mental hospitals. Acta Psychiatr Scand 57(5):361–368
Glen AI, Dodd M, Hulme EB, Kreitman N (1979) Mortality on lithium. Neuropsychobiology 5(3):167–173
Goldberg DP, Blackwell B (1970) Psychiatric illness in general practice. A detailed study using a new method of case identification. Br Med J [Clin Res] 2:439–442
Gottschalk LA, McGuire FL, Heiser JF, Dinovo EC (1979) A review of psychoactive drug-involved deaths in nine major United States cities. Int J Addict 14(6):735–758
Griesinger W (1865) Livre Y: curabilité et traitement des maladies mentales – section I: pronostic. In: Traité des maladies mentales. Pathologie et thérapeutique. Delahaye, Paris, pp 514–525
Gross G (1971) Etude de la longévité chez les malades mentaux. Arch Suisses Neurol Neurochir Psychiatrie 108(1):125–143
Hagnell O (1966) A prospective study of the incidence of mental disorder. Norstedts, Lund
Hall RC, Popkin MK, Stickney S (1978) Physical illness presenting as psychiatric disease. Arch Gen Psychiatry 35:1315–1320
Hermann P (1986) Les études de cohortes. In: Chanoit PF, Verbizier J (eds) Informatique et épidémiologie psychiatrique. Eres, Geneva, pp 167–187
Herridge CF (1960) Physical disorders in psychiatric illness. A study of 209 consecutive admissions. Lancet I:949–951
Hoenig J, Hamilton MW (1966) Mortality of psychiatric patients. Acta Psychiatr Scand 42(4):349–361
Hollister LE, Kosek JC (1965) Sudden death during treatment with phenothiazine derivatives. JAMA 192:1035–1038
Hussar AE (1962) Effect of tranquilizers on medical morbidity and mortality in a mental hospital. JAMA 179(9):682–686
Innes G, Millar WM (1970) Mortality among psychiatric patients. Scott Med J 15:143–148
Jameson MA, Shuman LJ, Young WW (1978) The effect of outpatient psychiatric utilisation of the costs of providing 3rd party coverage. Med Care 16:383
Johnson DA (1968) The evaluation of routine physical examination in psychiatric cases. Practitioner 200:696–697
Koranyi EK (1977) Fatalities in 2,070 psychiatric patients. Arch Gen Psychiatry 34:1137–1142
Koranyi EK (1979) Morbidity and rate of undiagnosed physical illnesses in a psychiatric clinic population. Arch Gen Psychiatry 36:414–419
Koskenvuo M, Sarna S, Kaprio J, Lonnqvist J (1979) Cause-specific mortality by marital status and social class in Finland during 1969–1971. Soc Sci Med 13A:691–697
Kramer M (1970) Les statistiques de santé mentale et leurs applications. WHO, Geneva
Lacrosse JM, Verhaegen L, Sand EA (1984) Analyse et évaluation critique du fonctionnement des secteurs psychiatriques en Belgique. OMS-WHO mental health services in pilot study areas, 3 vols. Ecole de Santé Publique, Université Libre de Bruxelles, Brussels

Leclerc A, Aiach P, Philippe A, Vennin M (1979) Morbidité, mortalité et classe sociale. Revue bibliographique portant sur divers aspects de la pathologie, et discussion. Rev Epidemiol Santé Publique 27(4):331–358

Maguire GP, Granville-Grossman KL (1968) Physical illness in psychiatric patients. Br J Psychiatry 115:1365–1369

Malzberg B (1953) Rates of discharge and rates of mortality among first admission to the New York civil state hospital (third paper). Ment Hyg 37:619–654

Niswander GD, Heslerud GM, Mitchel GD (1963) Changes in cause of death of psychiatric patients (a cross-sectional and longitudinal study over a 60-year period). Arch Gen Psychiatry 9:63–68

Ödegård Ö (1951) Mortality in Norwegian mental hospitals 1916–1941. Acta Genet (Basel) 11:141–173

Ödegård Ö (1952) The excess mortality of the insane. Acta Psychiatr Neurol Scand 27:353–367

Ödegård Ö (1967) Mortality in Norwegian psychiatric hospitals 1950–1962. Acta Genet (Basel) 17(1):137–153

Raymond L, Cochet B, Voinier B (1981) Sur mortalité en psychiatrie ambulatoire: premiers résultats d'une étude à Genève. Med Soc Prév Soz Präventiv Med 26:348–349

Ribourdouille MJ, Corten PF (1986) Mortalité chez des patients fréquentant un secteur psychiatrique. Acta Psychiatr Belg 86:514–525

Richardson HL, Graupner KI, Richardson ME (1966) Intramyocardial lesions in patients dying suddenly and unexpectedly. JAMA 195(4):254–260

Rorsman B (1974) Mortality among psychiatric patients. Acta Psychiatr Scand 50(3):354–375

Rorsman B, Hagnell O, Lanke J (1982) Mortality in the Lundby study (natural death in different forms of mental disorder in a total population investigated during a 25-year period). Neuropsychobiology 8:188–197

Ryan M (1982) Aspect of male mortality (USSR letter). Br Med J [ClinRes] 284:181–182

Salmon P, Sims ACP (1981) Smoking profiles of patients admitted for neurosis. Br J Psychiatry 139:43–46

Saugstad LF, Ödegård Ö (1979) Mortality in psychiatric hospitals in Norway 1950–1974. Acta Psychiatr Scand 59(4):431–447

Savino MT, Brody SA (1966) Discharge and death rates in California state hospitals: 1852–1954. Arch Gen Psychiatry 15:475–484

Selye H (1974) Stress sans détresse. La Presse, Montréal

Shepherd M (1957) A study of the major psychosis in an English County. Maudsley Monograph no 3, Oxford University Press, London

Shinozaki H (1976) An epidemiologic study of deaths of psychiatric inpatients. Compr Psychiatry 17:425–436

Sims ACP (1973) Mortality in neurosis. Lancet II:1072–1076

Sims ACP (1979) Discrimination between neurotics who die and neurotics who live. Acta Psychiatr Scand 59:317–325

Sims ACP (1984) Neurosis and mortality: investigating and association. J Psychosom Res 28(5):353–362

Sims ACP (1985) The hypothesis of an increased mortality associated with neurosis. IIIrd Congress of International Federation of Epidemiological Psychiatry, Sept 1985, Brussels, p 25

Sims ACP, Prior P (1978) The pattern of mortality in severe neuroses. Br J Psychiatry 133:299–305

Singer E, Garfinkel R, Cohen SM, Srole L (1976) Mortality and mental health: evidence from the Midtown Manhattan restudy. Soc Sci Med 10:517–525

Tefft BM, Pederson AM, Babigian HM (1977) Patterns of death among suicide attempters, a psychiatric population and a general population. Arch Gen Psychiatry 34:1155–61

Tokuhata GK, Stehman VA (1958) Mortality in state mental hospitals of Michigan 1950–1954. Public Health Rep 73:750–776

Tsuang MT, Woolson RF (1977) Mortality in patients with schizophrenia, mania, depression and surgical conditions. A comparison with general population mortality. Br J Psychiatry 130:162–166

Turunen S, Salminen J (1968) Neuroleptic treatment and mortality. Dis Nerv Syst 29(7):474–477

Von Bertalanffy L (1968) General system theory. Braziller, New York

von Krafft-Ebing R (1897) Chap II: mortalité – maladies intercurcurrentes importantes. In: Maloine (ed) Traité clinique de psychiatrie. Naloine, Paris, pp 263–268

Watkins Ch, Gilbert JE, Seale AL (1972) Causes of death in psychiatric hospitals. South Med J 65(8):969–975

Weiner B, Warvit RC (1977) Schizophrenia in Hawaii: analysis of cohort mortality risk in a multi-ethnic population. Br J Psychiatry 131:497–503

Westermeyer J (1978) Mortality and psychosis in a peasant society. J Nerv Ment Dis 166(11):769–774

WHO (1979) Myocardial infarction community register. Public health in Europe, 5. WHO, Copenhagen

Wood JB, Evenson RC, Chio DW, Hagan BJ (1985) Mortality variations among public mental health patients. Acta Psychiatr Scand 72:218–229

Zlotlow M, Paganini AE (1958) Fatalities in patients receiving chlorpromazine and reserpine during 1956–1957 at Pilgrim state hospital. Am J Psychiatry 115:154–156

Neurobiological Aspects of Psychiatric Consequences of Physical Illness

A. Carlsson

To try to translate the mental consequences of physical illness into the language of neurobiology is a fascinating though difficult and perhaps premature exercise. It should be obvious that when in moving from psychiatry to neurobiology, the dichotomy physical-mental, body-soul becomes rather awkward. To approach this problem in a serious way, it is necessary to try and locate the site in the brain that harbors the mind; many proposals concerning this location have been made in the past. To the extent that the site of the mind has been located, it must be concluded that any part of the organism that is outside this site must be defined as "body." This will probably include a considerable part of the brain itself, and therefore, from this point of view there are many brain disorders that are somatic. Epilepsy and Parkinson's disease, if not complicated by mental disturbances, would then be classified as "physical illness." The topic can be divided into two parts: in the first place, mental consequences of disease-related changes in blood chemistry, and second, mental changes caused by physical illness through other mechanisms.

Considering first the changes in blood chemistry that have to be considered in this context, these involve nutrients and metabolites, e.g., oxygen, carbon dioxide, inorganic irons including trace metals, pH changes, glucose, aminoacids, vitamins, etc. There are also hormones, many of which can modify mental functions quite substantially, as well as both endogenous toxic compounds. The possibility cannot be excluded that some mental disorders in the strict sense are indeed due to changes in blood chemistry. Some proposals along these lines have been proven correct, such as phenylketonuria and porphyria, but others have had to be rejected, such as hypotheses on the role of adrenochrome and "pink spot" in schizophrenia. The interesting possibility of aberrations in aminoacids and aminoacid availability as factors involved, e.g., in depression, panic disorder, and aggressive behavior is still under discussion.

In considering nerve-mediated influences, the possible consequences of pain and other distressing sensations on mental functions must be taken into account. Moreover, the very awareness of a disease, especially if it is chronic, disabling, and with a poor prognosis, may be of major importance; this is the psychogenic aspect of the problem. Regardless of the mechanism, there is enormous individual variation in the psychological response to physical ill-

Department of Pharmacology, University of Gothenburg, Box 33031, S-40033 Gothenburg

Interaction Between Mental and Physical Illness
Edited by R. Öhman et al.

ness, and this might even serve as a starting point for new therapeutic strategies. If the mechanisms underlying this variation could be understood new avenues for intervention might be found, in cases where this seems necessary. In this context, it must not be forgotten that illness does not necessarily have an altogether negative impact on the sick individual's mind. Sandblom (1983) has emphasized the apparently stimulating influence that physical as well as mental illness has exerted on the creativity of a large number of outstanding artists, philosophers, poets, scientists, etc. Dostojevski suffered from epilepsy and so did Mohammed – creative individuals indeed. Was Dostojevski an epileptic genius suffering from hypergraphia?

It is necessary to be open minded, when trying to approach the difficult problem of how painful and stressful experiences which are induced by physical illness can influence the human mind. To deal with this problem in neurobiological terms, the first thing is to try to envisage the human mind in such terms. Where is the mind located? Which part of the brain harbours it? As a starting point, one has to create some sort of a hypothetical model, drawn from knowledge in the realms of brain lesions, brain pathology, and drug effects. This knowledge may be expected to expand dramatically in the near future, given the imaging techniques that are now available or forthcoming.

A solid platform to build on would be the pharmacology of perhaps the most profound alteration of the human mind that is known – psychosis; here is much evidence that dopamine is involved in psychosis. It is known that psychotic behavior can be alleviated by a number of dopamine antagonists, either dopamine-depleting agents or dopamine receptor-blocking agents. We also know that psychotic behavior can be induced or aggravated by dopaminergic compounds, acting either directly on receptors or by releasing dopamine. If these receptors that are engaged in the alleviation or aggravation or induction of psychotic behavior could be located, we would know one site in the brain where a very important mental function is located.

Dopamine and its receptors can be detected in the human cortex, but the levels are very low indeed. It is interesting that they are lower than in other vertebrates, even in subhuman primates, so it seems as if in the evolutionary jump that has been taken from the subhuman primates to man, with its tremendous growth of the cortex, dopamine in the cortex has not evolved to the same extent. On the other hand, the striatum has indeed evolved along with the cortex, which points in the direction of striatal dopamine being considered in this context.

The highly simplified scheme in Fig. 1 may serve to illustrate this. What may have to be considered here is a number of negative feedback loops. From the cortex, there is a glutamate pathway to the striatum, which is excitatory. From the striatum to the thalamus, there is an inhibitory input. Classically, thalamus is considered as a relay station for many kinds of inputs from the external world to the cerebral cortex. It is now proposed that the thalamus serves as feedback controlled filter – controlled by the cortex through the striatum. The purpose of this filter might be to protect the cortex from an overload of

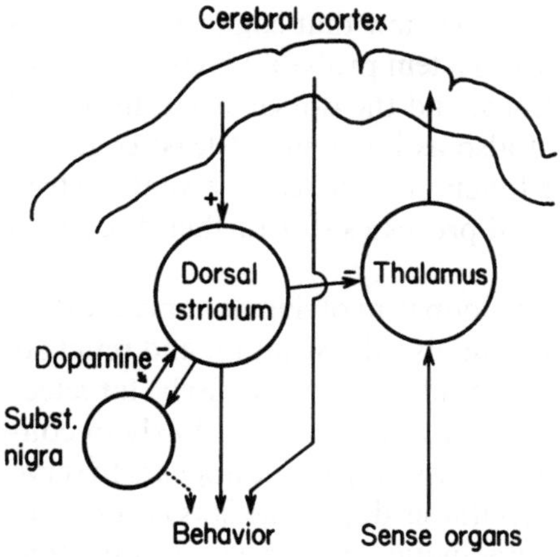

Fig. 1. Hypothetical corticostriatal, dopamine-modulated feedback loop controlling a thalamic sensory input filter. The dorsal striatum (caudate nucleus and putamen) receives a glutamatergic input from all parts of the neocortex, including the association areas of the frontal lobe. This input is excitatory. The dorsal striatum projects via the globus pallidus to the thalamus. The projection to the thalamus is inhibitory and serves to close the thalamic sensory input filter. The negative feedback loop thus obtained enables the cortex to protect itself from an overflow of sensory input. Moreover, the thalamic filter, part of which is precisely targeted, functions selectively to enable focussing on the most relevant input.

The feedback loop is modulated by the nigrostriatal dopamine pathway which is inhibitory on the striatum. An increased dopaminergic activity will thus open the thalamic filter.

Similarly, the ventral striatum receives an excitatory glutamatergic input from the limbic cortex and projects to the dorsomedial nucleus of the thalamus through an inhibitory pathway. Thus, a thalamic filter appears to exist also in the limbic system. The negative feedback loop thus obtained is modulated by the mesolimbic dopamine pathway, which is inhibitory on the ventral striatum and thus serves to open the thalamic filter. Both the dorsal and ventral striatum project, in addition to the thalamus, to the mesencephalic reticular formation by means of an inhibitory pathway.

The negative feedback loops obtained via the thalamic and mesencephalic reticular formations will enable the cortex to protect itself from hyperarousal. The modulation by means of the dopaminergic pathways will counteract the impact from the cortex and lead to increased arousal

information: it should be important for the cortex not to have more information than it can handle, since too much information could lead to confusion or various mental aberrations. On this negative feedback loop, there is a very important modulator: the dopaminergic nigrostriatal pathway which is inhibitory on the striatum. Thus, the glutamate and dopamine pathways antagonize and balance each other. To pursue the filter concept, an increased dopaminergic input would inhibit an inhibitory mechanism, which should lead to an opening up of the filter and to an increased flow of information to the cortex. According to recent mapping data, all parts of the cortex have inputs into the dorsal and/or ventral striatum, which probably means that all cortical functions are somehow regulated via either the dorsal or the ventral striatum. The frontal association areas have very strong inputs to the dorsal striatum, and there is also experimental evidence favoring the view that cognitive functions are under striatal control. Thus, this control system probably involves all cortical functions, including cognitive functions, and the dorsal striatum should be looked upon not merely as motor but also as involving at least cognitive functions also. It probably has still other functions, whereas the ventral striatum may be involved in affective, emotional processes (for further discussion and references, see Carlsson 1988).

There seem to be several similar feedback loops, involving not only the dorsal and ventral striatum and the thalamus, but also the striatum and reticular formation. Those involving the thalamus could be very precisely targeted, whereas those involving the reticular formation would be more likely to control a general arousal mechanism. In all these cases, dopamine appears to serve as a modulator. Thus, according to this hypothesis dopamine acts as a modulator in a rather similar way both for motor activities and for a variety of mental functions. These filters could be looked upon in a grossly quantitative manner: it could be said that the filter is either opened up or closed, but it could also be much more sophisticated. To account for the affective aspects, there could be filters related to the punishment and reward system. Thus, mania might be due to a widely open filter, leading to a very high input, emphasizing the reward aspects, which in turn should lead to a considerable output. Depression could be the other way round, with the filter more or less closed. To pursue the analogy further, it could be said that the filter also serves as a lens, and that this lens could be either regular or give a very distorted picture of the environment, and that leads into the area of schizophrenia.

Conclusion

It should be emphasized again that the reaction to physical illness shows a tremendous individual variation. This could be due to the setting of the internal circuit discussed above. Thus, the depression, anxiety, asthenia, etc. which are induced by physical illness might well respond to pharmacological treatment which aims to manipulate this circuitry. It may be that this is in fact being done already. This approach can no doubt be improved as more is learned about the physiology and pharmacology of the relevant circuitry in the brain.

References

Carlsson A (1988) Speculations on the control of mental and motor functions by dopamine-modulated cortico-striato-thalamo-cortical feedback loops. Mount Sinai J Med 55:6–10

Sandblom Ph (1983) Skapande och sjukdom. Fingraf, Södertälje

On the State of Knowledge in Neurobiological Psychiatry

R. Fog

Our present knowledge of neurobiological mechanisms in psychosomatic disorders or in mental disturbances connected with physical illness is practically nil. This reflects the state of knowledge in biological psychiatry as a whole, where we have many theories, some circumstantial evidence, but few facts. This situation influences many aspects of psychiatry, of which the following are some.

Classifications

It has been almost impossible to reach a reasonable consensus in defining psychosomatic disorders. Syndromes are often talked about as "anxiety," "depression," or "asthenia" (Ottoson, this volume), but it must be realized that these vague terms are only describing symptoms, which again are ill-defined. Asthenia is a term parallel to coughing, which may be a result of many different underlying biological causes.

Neurobiological Substrates

There is a fairly good knowledge of brain mechanisms involved in respiration, blood pressure, etc., whereas nearly nothing is known of brain mechanisms involved in thinking, feeling, and other higher functions. "The limbic system" and "the extrapyramidal system" are discussed (Carlsson, this volume), but it must be admitted that we are operating in too simplistic terms. However, more knowledge is coming forward concerning brain mechanisms in reward and punishment (Ashton 1987), whilst theories of the interactions between striatal, thalamic, and cortical functions (Carlsson, this volume) seem promising.

Animal Models

There is a great need in psychiatric research for better animal models. Most animal studies are made with rodents, but it is a disturbing fact that even our

Laboratory of Psychopharmacology, St. Hans Hospital, DK-4000 Roskilde

Interaction Between Mental and Physical Illness
Edited by R. Öhman et al.

closest "cousins," the gorilla and the orangutan, conduct very different social lives from us, and neither of these have any language – both things of great importance in psychiatric "modelling."

Hypotheses

We are trying to establish hypotheses and models of psychiatric diseases by comparing different pathological states. Temporal lobe epilepsy (Bolwig, this volume) may be a model for schizophrenia, and so may the amphetamine psychosis (Fog 1972). The analogies are, however, weakened by the doubt, shared now by many researchers, as to whether schizophrenia is in fact a diagnostic entity. The involvement of dopamine in antipsychotic effects is still the best-established fact concerning brain mechanisms in schizophrenic symptomatology. Just the same could be said, however, of other psychiatric and neurological disorders such as Parkinsonism, Huntington's chorea, Tourette's syndrome, and mania (Fog and Regeur 1986). This may not be very surprising, since dopaminergic areas in the basal ganglia represent the "output system" for a large number of brain functions. Influencing dopamine seems, therefore, to be the safest way of obtaining an effect upon a whole range of neuropsychiatric diseases (Fog and Regeur 1986).

The dopamine hypothesis is almost exclusively based upon circumstantial evidence from pharmacology. The PET scan technique (Carlsson, this volume) adds to our knowledge, but it has to be admitted that even the most potent antidopaminergic drug has no curable effect upon schizophrenic symptoms. It is necessary, therefore, in connection with dopamine to study other brain mechanisms and other neurotransmitters such as glutamate, GABA, acetylcholine, and peptide (Scheel-Krüger and Arnt 1986).

Aetiology and Pathogenesis

The principle of influencing pathogenetic factors has been very successful in medicine, whereas attempts at finding etiological factors have been disappointing. Diabetes is a very good example of this. It has therefore been suggested that instead of seeking for root causes of disorder, psychiatrists should search for maximally effective intervention (Beahrs 1986).

Some investigations seem to suggest an influence of psychological factors on the course of even a cancerous disease (Häfner, this volume). Psychotherapy is suggested in some of these cases, but it should be remembered that our remarkable ignorance concerning the actual effectiveness of psychoanalysis and psychotherapy still persists, well into the last decades of this century (Clare 1984). There must be great care taken in the analyzing of data from these investigations; and it should not be forgotten that general paralysis was earlier considered a reactive psychosis. Even when its relationship to the syphilis bacteria was demonstrated, the psychosis was still regarded for some years as a reaction to a sinful behavior.

Psychopharmacological Treatment

No drugs are really effective in treating psychosomatic disorders. The drugs most commonly used are benzodiazepines, antidepressants, and (small doses of) neuroleptics. These drugs have very different profiles of action, and it seems impossible to get any hints of brain pathology from these pharmacological data. All the drugs have some "psychosedative" effects, and this may be seen in the light of the theories of filter mechanisms of the brain (Carlsson, this volume).

It is not easy to suggest future strategies for research: most effective drug treatments in psychiatry have been found by pure coincidence. One logical way suggested by Schou (Fog 1986) is to study different effective somatic treatments (in depression, e.g., cyclic antidepressants, MAO inhibitors, ECT, lithium) and look for common neurobiological mechanisms. Modern brain imaging techniques (Carlsson, this volume) and further biochemical studies will undoubtedly bring us more knowledge of pathogenetic factors in psychiatric disorders.

References

Ashton H (1987) Brain systems, disorders and psychotropic drugs. Oxford University Press, Oxford
Beahrs JO (1986) Limits of scientific psychiatry. Brunner-Mazel, New York
Clare AW (1984) Psychotherapy. In: Duncan R, Weston-Smith M (eds) The encyclopedia of medical ignorance. Pergamon, Oxford, pp 1–7
Fog R (1972) On stereotypy and catalepsy. Acta Neurol Scand 48 [Suppl 50]:1–66
Fog R (1986) An overview of neurobiological factors in antidepressant treatment. Acta Pharmacol Toxicol 56 [Suppl 1]:212–214
Fog R, Regeur L (1986) Neuropharmacology of tics. Rev Neurol (Paris) 142:856–859
Scheel-Krüger J, Arnt J (1986) New aspects on the role of dopamine, acetylcholine and GABA in the development of tardive dyskenesia. In: Casey DE, Chase TN, Christensen AV, Gerlach (eds) Dyskinesia, research and treatment. Springer, Berlin Heidelberg New York, pp 46–57

Psychosocial and Psychosomatic Aspects of AIDS Research

M. ERMANN

Against a background of experiences in psychosomatic medicine and psychotherapy, this paper will elaborate the general aspects of research in AIDS and HIV infections. It will not discuss the neuropathological aspects, and especially the important neurotropic functions of the infection.

Development of the HIV-AIDS Problem Within the Psychosocial and Psychosomatic Framework

Since AIDS was first identified in Europe at the beginning of the 1980s, it has become clear that the HIV-AIDS problem has very great psychosocial and psychosomatic implications (Coates et al. 1984; Joseph et al. 1984; Rubinow 1985). From the beginning, some basic facts became clear which showed the psychosocial dimension of the problem. AIDS and HIV infections have been – at least at the beginning – associated with homosexuality, drug use, imprisonment, and hemophilia. As a consequence, the AIDS problem has been related to preexisting handicaps. The patients have to cope either with sexual deviation and minority problems, with chronic mental illness and social stress, or with chronic somatic disease and possibly social isolation. There is therefore a coincidence of infection and preexisting psychosocial stress (Forstein 1984), so that supporting the patient and increasing his coping ability is assumed to be an important factor in relation to the course of the disease.

Coping with the preexisting problems has been handicapped by prejudice and isolation of those subgroups in which the majority of cases have appeared (Morin and Batchelor 1984). Society identified homosexuals especially as the high risk group and neglected the important difference between risk group and risk behavior. Thereby, the psychological situation in this minority group worsened and, for a long time, the risk behavior of heterosexuals was neglected.

Individual patients have been isolated because of infection fears, which were partially irrational; family relationships and friendships have been handicapped, and families affected as a whole. Instead of making use of social and psychological support, the patients have withdrawn with guilt feelings and

Abteilung für Psychotherapie und Psychosomatik der Universitäts-Nervenklinik, Nußbaumstraße 7, 8000 München 2

Interaction Between Mental and Physical Illness
Edited by R. Öhman et al.

fear. These individual and family anxieties and distress have been augmented by isolation, by practical disadvantages, and by discrimination. The conditions for coping with HIV infection and AIDS have thereby been impaired (Fisher 1986).

The more the risk behavior especially in the sexual field was identified, the more it became obvious that the most effective means of prevention is to be health education and counselling. Changing sexual risk behavior and drug use became a most important strategy, but this involves self-understanding – not only within the homosexual and bisexual groups. It became obvious that the efficiency of anti-AIDS campaigns is dependent on complex motivational factors, which are largely unknown. Therefore, the effects and side-effects of political preventive measures have come under discussion (Temoshok et al. 1987).

AIDS phobia has become an increasing problem. Its resulting problems are irrational sexual anxieties and restrictive sexual practices, with all their consequences to mental health. All these developments have caused increasing consciousness of the psychosocial aspects of the AIDS problem (Cassens 1985). The need for psychosocial and psychosomatic research has been emphasized by most AIDS programs, although up to now – 1987 – there has been relatively little activity in this area, or financial support for it. Within the scientific literature, most papers deal with the clinical problems of psychiatric consultation, symptomatology, and psychotherapeutic interventions. There are few reports from research programs and almost no representative results.

Present Situation

Since blood transfusion is no longer risk-bound, three types of linear risk behavior have to be differentiated (Green and Müller 1986):

1. Changing of sexual partners, homosexual as well as heterosexual
2. Injection of drugs
3. Prostitution

During the past two years, a development has taken place within the high-risk groups (Emmons et al. 1986). This line of development will be discussed with special reference to the City of Munich (Görgens et al. 1987; Ermann et al. 1988), as observed from contacts with the local health and self-care services there.

Among *hemophiliacs*, it can be assumed that no further contagion is generally taking place. Seroconversion in this group was due to factor substitution before 1985. In Germany, seropositive patients represent more than half the clients of hemostasiology centers. The problem of these patients is how to cope with the risk of AIDS and how to deal with their sexuality. From the point of view of research, the incidence of AIDS and related syndromes is of special interest. Some clinicians believe that the incidence within hemophiliacs is smaller than within seropositive homosexuals and drug users, but up to now, no exact data are available on this question. If this assumption is corroborated, the important questions arise – what are the reasons for these differences, and especially, what are the protective factors?

Unfortunately, an invisible boundary has to be overcome between hemophiliacs and other risk groups. Therefore, obtaining control groups is an important practical problem of research in this area.

The second risk groups are *homosexual and bisexual men*: they appear to have basically changed their sexual behavior. The available information about risks, and especially about unsafe anal intercourse, has broadly been adopted by them, and safer sex is accepted as the essential means of prevention. In spite of this hopeful aspect, this group remains one of the most exposed risk groups for new infection as well as the manifestation of AIDS. Therefore, the central tasks of research in relation to this group are:

1. To further increase compliance with preventive advice
2. To further modify sexual behavior
3. To support patients' coping skills with the contagion
4. To prevent the manifestation of AIDS
5. To support methods of dealing with the manifest illness

As prevention is the most effective approach, and since unsafe anal intercourse has turned out to play by far the most important role as a means of contamination, the most topical research area should be to investigate the psychosocial and social implications of AIDS. We would take a small step forward if we had a better knowledge of the conditions which facilitate unsafe anal intercourse among informed homosexuals, if we had a better insight into both the conscious and unconscious motives for doing so, and if we had predictors for behavioral change (Emmons et al. 1986).

Among other factors, agression appears to be one of the crucial psychodynamic motives, and it would no doubt be worth studying the interaction between aggression and compliance with psychosocial advice.

The more prevention can become effective, the more research will center around the problems of dealing with a life-threatening illness. In this complex area, some orientation might be obtained from psychosomatic research in other chronic diseases, especially cancer, myocardial infarction, and perhaps tuberculosis, though the parallel seems to be limited to general coping processes. The specific problem in the HIV infection is that the psychosocial cofactors of the change from the premorbid state to the AIDS disease are unknown and there is no proven knowledge about preventive factors.

Questions which need to be answered include: What is the influence of helplessness, anxiety, depression, aggression, and social fear on "illness behavior" and on the course of the disease? What is the effect of a health-conscious lifestyle, of problem-solving groups, and of self-help activities? What influence have professional psychosocial counselling and psychotherapeutic interventions? These are but the most urgent of the questions with tremendous relevance to psychosocial care.

The third risk group are *intravenous drug users* (Ramloch-Sohl and Wiederkehr 1986). These patients seem to be the outsiders of AIDS care and research, except for the small group which is sufficiently integrated into drug rehabilitation programs. The general problems are lack of acceptance of psychosocial advice, of information, and of insight and compliance with respect to behavioral change. Contamination by drug injections, combined with prostitution, will probably be the most important danger for new HIV contagions in the future. The most important approach for research in this group seems to be the identification of factors which might increase compliance. A change of addictive behavior is essential: oral substitution must be considered, in the absence of better alternatives. But at this point, research becomes involved with political measures, in a field of the highest priority. Researchers' suggestions for health prevention have to be based on objective investigations but, on the other hand, the effect of health policy measures has to be evaluated on the basis of rational research.

The second area of research on drug addicts is the discovery of psychosocial cofactors which influence the progress of the illness. Some factors are being investigated, but have not been conclusively demonstrated to be relevant. These include:

1. The immunosuppressive effect of the drugs, which is also assumed to be responsible for the onset and progress of hepatitis in addicts
2. The psychological stress of addiction and the poor lifestyle centered around obtaining and consuming drugs
3. The permanent conflicts related to prostitution

Studies comparing addicts with other risk groups are needed to obtain more detailed knowledge and more refined hypotheses about the impact of psychosocial stress or the addicts' social situation.

The third problem is how to deal with contagion and illness. Addicts tend to neglect symptoms. They refuse advice about a more healthy way of life, such as simple preventive measures against reinfection or secondary infection, and towards stabilization. These problems are based on the disorder of the personality, which is related to their drug problems. The coincidence of addiction, prostitution, contamination, and AIDS manifestation in addicts is generally more a social problem than a psychological one.

The last group has become of increasing importance in recent years: *heterosexuals with multiple sexual partners*. In spite of information campaigns, knowledge about the risk of AIDS is insufficient in this group. Projection and denial lead to a misinterpretation of AIDS as a homosexual disease, and consequently, sexual behavior shows little change. The most important factor seems to be prejudice against safer sex and especially against condoms: it is a vital question to find predictors for better compliance and advice about this (Sherr 1987; Temoshok et al. 1987). Their individual problems of coping and dealing with the contagion are in general equivalent to those of homosexuals. An additional problem which arises in married heterosexuals is the impact of the infection on the partnership and on the family. Little experience about these problems has been reported in the literature up to now.

Areas of Needed Research

Some work is being done within all these areas, though AIDS research in general centers around biological problems, especially virology and immunology. The problem of psychosocial and psychosomatic research is that these require new models of collaboration, which means more than merely adding social and psychological variables to biological approaches.

The first urgent area is investigation of *psychosocial cofactors* and *preventive factors* in HIV infection and the manifestation of AIDS. Since the onset of the problem, the investigation of cofactors and preventive factors has been under discussion. The leading idea is to find out why not all individuals with a risk behavior develop a seroconversion, and why certain seropositive persons develop AIDS and related syndromes sooner than others. The principal hypothesis is that in addition to biological factors, psychological variables influence susceptibility to the HIV infection and the course of the disease, especially at the onset of the manifestation of AIDS. In this area, psychoimmunological approaches are needed to determine specific host factors and mediator mechanisms. Probably research in cancer (Cohen et al. 1982) and in other infections may help to find plausible hypotheses. The following factors are currently under discussion.

1. General psychosocial stress: social isolation, social fear, and lack of social support. In this connection, it should be mentioned that there is the possibility that political preventive measures might put additional pressure on the patients in question.
2. A more specific approach is needed to find out predictors from the wide range of psychosocial factors, e.g., helplessness, hopelessness, aggression, anxiety, depression, and ego weakness. The change of preexisting coping mechanisms by the infection and manifestation of AIDS needs to be studied, as well as the influence of preexisting neurotic conflicts and psychotic disorders.

From the psychodynamic point of view, the impact of specific structural conflicts on the course of the disease should be investigated. From the behavioral point of view, the hypotheses of conditioning immunosuppressive processes needs to be examined within the special group of HIV-infected patients. In this area of specific psychosocial cofactors, prospective studies and studies of those who escape infection are needed.

The second urgent area of research is on *coping* and *illness progress*. Here, a broad approach to threatening and chronic diseases may provide a basic orientation. Presumptive cofactors like ego strength, capacity for problem solving, self-competence, insight, availability of family support, and lack of secondary psychosomatic disturbances should be investigated. In our own project, we are examining the hypothesis that illness onset is associated with failure of coping mechanisms because of individual neurotic conflicts.

The third area is the *psychology of risk behavior*. Here, some orientation may be provided by compliance research. The distinction between compliers and noncompliers should be investigated. Likely cofactors are adoption of information and availability of alternatives. Special interest should be given to confidence and anxiety which may arise from institutional interactions in medical and psychosocial care and from administrative measures, as well as to the effect of fear-based preventive campaigns.

The fourth and perhaps most urgent area is the *evaluation of psychosocial and psychotherapeutic interventions*. The crucial point is to objectify the effects of different intervention strategies on the psychosocial and medical status and on illness-related aspects of behavior. The most exciting perspective is to find out specific influences of psychotherapeutic interventions on the course of the biological progress of the disease. It could be exciting to prove that psychological interventions with regard to the neurotic personality structure and conflicts are able to prevent the AIDS manifestation in seropositive persons. Perhaps this is a vision of the future. But what we need urgently today is to find out which interventions really do effect changes of behavior, which means behavior with regard to risk and health-damaging attitudes.

References

Cassens BJ (1985) Social consequences of AIDS. Ann Intern Med 103:768–771

Coates TJ, Temoshok L, Mander J (1984) Psychosocial research is necessary to understanding and treating of AIDS. Am Psychol 39:1309–1314

Cohen J, Cullen JW, Martin LR (eds) (1982) Psychosocial aspects of cancer. Raven, New York

Emmons CA, Joseph JG, Kessler RC, Wortman CB, Montgomery SB, Ostrow DG (1986) Psychosocial predictors of reported behavior change in homosexual men at risk for AIDS. Health Educ Q 13:331–345

Ermann M, Garwers C, Hutner G, Scheil A, Schneider MM, Seidl O, Zippel S (1988) Psychosocial HIV/AIDS-care (in German). Munch Med Wochenschr 130:15–18

Fisher EJ (1986) Consider the psychosocial consequences of AIDS. Mich Med J 85:95–96

Forstein M (1984) The psychosocial impact of AIDS. Semin Oncol 11:77–82

Görgens K, Kathke N, Krahnke H (1987) Psychosocial problems, health education and behavioral changes of sexual practices and HIF infection (in German). AIDS-Forschung (AIFO) 2:171–175

Green J, Müller D (1986) AIDS, the story of the disease. Grafton, London

Joseph JG, Emmons CA, Keller RC, Wortman CB, O'Brien K, Hocker WT, Schaefer C (1984) Coping with the threat of AIDS. Am Psychol 39:1297–1302

Morin SF, Batchelor WF (1984) Responding to the psychological crisis of AIDS. Public Health Rep 99:4–9

Ramlock-Sohl M, Wiederkehr P (1986) AIDS and its problems for drug care professionals (in German). AIDS-Forschung (AIFO) 1:328–335

Rubinow DR (1985) Psychological impacts of AIDS. In: Wolcott DL et al. (eds) AIDS and consultation liaison psychiatry. Gen Hosp Psychiatry 7:280–292

Sherr L (1987) An evaluation of the UK government health education campaign on Aids. Psychol Health 1:61–72

Temoshok L, Sweet DM, Zich J (1987) A three city comparison of the public's knowledge and attitude about AIDS. Psychol Health 1:43–60

Psychiatric Consequences of High Technology in Medical Care

P. Tienari

The definition of high technology must be arbitrary, because some of today's high technology may become tomorrow's low technology, just as some of today's research becomes tomorrow's routine. The definition might also include complexity and costliness, which result in restricted availability, usually in a limited number of localities and under the control of specialist staff. It follows from this that the demand for the use high technology exceeds the supply, so that some form of explicit rationing is required. It is possible to analyse high technology according to the type of machine or instrument used: radiological, endoscopic, anesthetic, etc. But the debate concerns less the mechanics than the secondary consequences which the increasing use of high technology may have on the practice of medicine, both in general and for particular patients. Consideration is required as to where high technology fits into the agenda of the medical task. However, in order to analyze its potential contribution to the medical task, as well as its secondary influences, it is useful to identify activities separately and to itemize the main types of action involved in each of these steps (Jennet 1984).

Even with all the modern therapeutic advances, cure is a possible objective in only a minority of the patients diagnosed as having a condition that will not resolve spontaneously. Even in such cases, cure is seldom absolutely certain, and intervention usually involves some risks of complication. Most of the patients now admitted to hospital suffer from progressive diseases, the ultimate outcome of which cannot be influenced, but it is an oversimplification to describe the needs of these patients as care, and then to contrast that with cure. Rescue procedures are often successful in postponing death, and they sometimes result in cure. In most cases, they prolong the survival of disabled patients, but sometimes the quality of life of these people is much worse after the rescue than it was before the crisis. Rescue procedures include intensive care, renal dialysis and transplantation, much open heart and neonatal surgery, and a good deal of treatment for cancer. Rescue usually involves high technology.

A distinction must therefore be made between high technology per se and the different ways in which it is used: much of the criticism of technology is fuelled by the inappropriate application of tools that have considerable poten-

Department of Psychiatry, University of Oulu, SF-90210 Oulu

Interaction Between Mental and Physical Illness
Edited by R. Öhman et al.

tial benefit, if they are properly employed. Most of the tools of medical technology can be regarded as fullfilling one of the five technological tasks. These are: visualising parts of the body, measuring physiological function, substituting lost functions, contributing to surgical procedures, and processing information.

This classification of medical technology by function may be useful for analytical purposes, but in practice, the tools of technology take their place alongside the traditional procedures. Nonetheless, there are certain medical activities which involve so much technology that they are immediately recognizable as high-technology packages, e.g., intensive care, renal dialysis and transplantation, and open-heart surgery. Some specialties, such as obstetrics and neurosurgery, have certain high-technology components, but retain much traditional activity, while others, such as radiology and laboratory medicine, are almost completely technological. In patient-contact technologies, reference is often made to the contrast between invasive and noninvasive techniques. Views will differ as to what constitutes an invasive technique, but one objective of technological development is to achieve safer and less invasive methods – a goal already reached in many areas.

Changes in the practice and organization of medicine in the past quarter of a century have fundamentally altered the role of hospital doctors, particularly those whose specialty involves the use of high-technology medicine. No one can provide complex services of this kind without the assistance of a team of other specially trained staff, nor can he prescribe expensive service on his own authority: this is because the supply of such services inevitably requires some form of explicit or implicit rationing. The availability of such technology is limited, both because of its cost and because even if money were no problem, there would not be enough skilled staff to meet the demand. The doctor is no longer a solitary provider, making a personal social contact with the patient. Rather, he has become a member of a large team that includes other doctors, technicians, and administrators – in addition to his traditional team mate, the nurse.

When diagnostic technology reveals disease, there is often a too ready assumption that effective treatment will logically ensue; campaigns for early detection of disease, particularly cancer, have sometimes resulted in doctors becoming victims of their own propaganda. Unfortunately, the evidence that early diagnosis results in improved outcome is still limited to relatively few instances. The early diagnosis of an untreatable disease may do no more than prolong the period of worry for the patient and the family. Much of the debate concerning our therapeutic technology is about its failures, which in fact result largely from its use on patients who either do not benefit at all from it, or who derive only temporary improvement, or whose rescue leaves them more severely disabled than they were originally.

A more general complaint against technological monitoring is that it may seem to distance the patient from his doctors and nurses, that it reduces the comfort of contact, the time for talk. Staff may indeed be tempted to glance at the machine displays and forget to say anything to the patient, who is denied even the physical touching involved in taking the pulse. Intensive care units may even have central consoles where nurses scan banks of television screens showing the parameters of many patients, sometimes even their faces. However, talking is no triviality: it is the most important single thread running through the relationship between doctor and patient or nurse and patient. But talk is a demanding task; it takes time, and time costs money. In hospital, high technology should relieve the doctor and the nurse of the time-consuming course of writing longhand notes and charts, of filling forms, and taking repeated observations by hand and eye. That ought to mean more time for talking to patients.

As components or ancillary factors in the technological revolution, doctors are witnessing (Rosch and Kearney 1985):

1. The ongoing computerization of medicine via increasingly sophisticated diagnostic and therapeutic instrumentation, which contribute to a depersonalisation of the patient.
2. A boom of new theory and design in computerized techniques which the doctor must keep abreast of, with resulting decrease in the time available for patient care.
3. A trend toward specialization and subspecialization in medicine and a compartmentalization of patient care, which increases the quantity of medical care in terms of specialists seen, diagnostic procedures performed, and various blood tests administered, but impairs the quality of direct doctor-patient personal interaction.
4. A reimbursement system which recognizes only procedural services, but not cognitive skills, thereby paying the doctor for doing something to his patient – surgery, X-rays, blood tests, etc. Remuneration is based on objective services, which can be quantified and assigned a specific monetary value, but not for subjective services such as listening, counseling, empathy, or caring.

At times, the effective treatment of an illness requires special equipment, special arrangements, and specially trained personnel, and it has been found useful to concentrate these in specialized wards. At the same time, however, it has become obvious that maximum efficiency in observing and treating somatic illness may also involve factors which are seriously adverse to the patient's psychological condition.

Radiotherapy is one of the more recently developed tools of medicine. The fact that radiation cannot be directly detected lends a particularly terrifying quality to radiotherapy as perceived by the patients – a quality not associated with more tangible and sensorily observable procedures. This terrifying aspect is emphasized by the patient's loneliness during the therapy: he is left alone with the huge apparatus, in a situation where nothing seems to happen, but which is so dangerous that nobody dares to be in the same room with him. Precisely because radiotherapy is difficult to understand and because radioactivity is generally known to be dangerous, this therapy tends to evoke anxious questions and fantasies in the patient.

In one study, 200 cancer patients were analyzed, half of whom received betathrone therapy and half linear accelerator therapy. The linear accelerator is a relatively small machine with quiet operation, and the daily treatment takes 2–3 min. The betathrone, on the other hand, is a very large and extremely loud machine, and the daily treatment takes 15–20 min. The incidence and severity of anxiety and depression were high in both groups, but as radiotherapy continued, these symptoms tended to decrease in intensity among the patients treated with the linear accelerator and to increase among the betathrone patients. The patients who denied knowledge of their diagnosis were initially less depressed and remained less depressed than those who knew or suspected they had cancer (Forester et al. 1978).

The technical developments of recent decades have made it possible to keep patients alive for shorter or longer periods by means of mechanical contrivances. The cardiac pacemaker is an example of a device that maintains and protects a vital function; Crisp and Stonehill (1969) found that the patients with an external pacemaker were much more anxious and depressed than those with an internal one. The former also had more fears, realistic as well as unrealistic, that something might happen to the device. It is obvious that external placement makes it harder for the patient to forget his dependence on the pacemaker and to integrate it into his body image than internal placement, where the pacemaker is out of sight.

Patients requiring repeated dialysis regularly suffer from depression of varying severity, and loss of social contacts is also common, especially among single patients. Chronic hemodialysis is stressful for the patient: the main sources of stress are the restrictions, the dependency, the patient's own increased aggression, the changes in body image, and the threat of death. Patients handle this stressful situation by mobilizing their defences, including denial, isolation, reaction formation, and displacement, as well as by introjection and projection. Though major psychiatric complications are rare, depression is found in about half the patients, and anxiety in one-third. Chronic hemodialysis is also stressful for the staff, and leads to frustrations and a high level of aggression among its members (DeNour and Kaplan 1976).

Advances in public health and in the medical treatment of acute disease have the consequence of increasing the incidence of chronic conditions, which often require long-term observance of major limitations of personal habits and even lifestyle. For the patient on chronic hemodialysis, maintenance of life and health depends on his adjustment to restrictions of diet and fluid intake that are stringent and difficult to maintain. It is not surprising that noncompliance with these restrictions has been widely reported, and is the focus of much attention.

Previous life adjustment and capacity for self-restraint have been identified as predictors of good adjustment, whereas anxiety, depression, hostility, and somatic complaints have been found to be predictive of poor adjustment. Adolescents have a greater problem, through having to deal with two kinds of stresses at the same time – maturational difficulties and dialysis – both involving dependency conflicts. They may experience an uncertain body image, be moody and uncooperative, and generally pose difficulties for the dialysis staff, who tend to be over-protective with this group (Gonsalves-Ebrahim et al. 1987).

Steidl et al. (1980) examined the relationships between compliance with the medical condition and family functioning, in patients on dialysis; they used a fairly reliable family assessment tool (Beavers-Timberlawn Family Evaluation Scales), in which family interactions are rated from a 30-min videotape. It was found that overall family functioning was significantly associated with the medical condition, and that specific components of family functioning (strong coalition between parents, close family relationships that respect individuality, and warm affectionate mood) were associated with compliance.

Depression is the condition most likely to threaten all the patients who depend on mechanical devices. As in all dependence relationships, dependence on a machine tends to encourage regression and the giving up of adult functioning and relationships. Although counteracting regression, depression, and passivity is the doctor's central task in dealing with all chronic patients, the patient's dependence on mechanical contrivances generally requires special support for the adult and active elements of his personality.

Intensive care units are specialized units with trained staff and special equipment to suit the needs of the patients. They have developed as a result of medical specialization and technology and have served as laboratories for the study of the behavior of patients and staff during a critical phase of illness. Attention was directed to these units because of the frequently disruptive behavior and experiences of both patients and staff. During the 1960s, a number of studies indicated that psychosis developed in 38%–70% of the patients recovering from open-heart surgery. In typical cases, the psychosis begins only 3–4 days after the operation and is characterized by delusions, disorientation, and often paranoia. Postulating the causes of such developments, Kornfeld (1972) noted that the patients were forced into virtual immobility by the postoperative pains, as well as by the various wires and tubes (EEG, drip, catether); they were continuously exposed to the flickering oscilloscopes of the electronic monitors and the endless hissing and humming of their oxygen tent. Alarming sounds were occasionally heard from the neighboring beds, staff kept coming and going, and the lights were on day and night. The conclusion was reached that the arrangement of the recovery room created an environment combining two factors that are well-known experimentally as causing psychosis – sensory monotony and sleep deprivation. Kornfeld et al. (1965) also identified such responses as anxiety, frustrations, sadness, anger, and fatigue in the staff.

Kimball's (1979) attention was first directed towards the process he observed in the patients, and later to the interactions between staff and patients, and staff and staff. He concluded that patients' experiences often led at first to illusions and subsequently to delusions and hallucinations, as part of an altered state of consciousness. It was his observation that the very designation of "craziness" served to put a greater distance between the patient and his environment, as more anxiety was aroused in the intensive care unit staff and in the patient's relatives. This behavior by the staff and family further isolated and alienated the patient, diminishing communication and even the frequency of medical contacts. As time and their research proceeded, it became more and more apparent that the discomfort in the patient was not so much of the disease as of his response to the experience of illness, the environment, and those within it.

Cassem and Hackett (1971) have identified a pattern of emotional response which is fairly characteristic of patients surviving an acute myocardial infarction in an intensive care unit. From the onset of the infarct, as measured in the hospital, anxiety mounts, peaking by the second day. It is directly correlated with the intensity and extent of the symptoms, notably pain. Anxiety is partially warded off by denial, which may relate to the fact of illness, its severity, its treatment, and especially the feeling of being ill; the behavioral counterpart of anxiety and denial is often impulsiveness. Anxiety gives way to what the authors call depression, which could also be called sadness, rising to a peak by the fourth day and thereafter dropping off; the patient fights against depression, using his characteristic defences.

Cardiac surgery was started with closed mitral commissurotomy, which was later followed by open-heart surgery, primarily of valvular and congenital defects, and most recently, coronary artery bypass grafting. It has been said that the next decade will probably witness the further development of artificial hearts and progress in transplantation. While the specific cardiac operations may have changed, an understanding of the patient's personality profiles and motivations for surgery continues to have relevance as a predictor of the clinical outcome.

Kimball (1977) placed the patients preoperatively into four categories, in an attempt to predict the operative and postoperative course. "Adjusted" patients were psychologically healthy and realistic; "symbiotic" patients were illness-dependent; "anxious" patients, although denying anxiety, showed it in their behavior. "Depressed" patients had "given in" and then "given up", and were poorly motivated for surgery. The adjusted patients did best 15 months later, with three-quarters of them having had a benign recovery. The symbiotic patients, on the other hand, had prolonged convalescence and a poor outcome, with only 7% rated as improved. The anxious patients had a 25% surgical mortality, often with arrhythmias, and a variable outcome, while the depressed patients fared the worst, with a 70% death rate and poor outcome for the survivors.

In the Oulu open-heart surgery study, the pre-operative estimate of prognosis was most successful in the group with no post-operative psychiatric complications. It was also found that the subjects who developed a psychiatric complication immediately after the operation had been estimated by a psychiatrist, 1 or 2 days before the operation, to be more anxious than the subjects without complications. After 17 months, it turned out that those with poor recovery had considered the time to prepare for the operation too short, thought their own attitude towards the treatment was of no significance, and had expressed less dissatisfaction with the treatment during its whole course. The psychiatrist had evaluated their tolerance of stress to be worse than that of the others' (in the pre-operative interview). Those with a good recovery after 12 months had been more satisfied with themselves before the operation, while the psychiatrist had estimated their prognosis to be better in the pre-operative interview, and their coping ability (use of defences) more adequate than in the case of the others. They had also reported a better social adjustment and more pleasure in their human relationships in the pre-operative interview (Tienari et al. 1983).

It seems likely that clinical methods may help to identify pre-operatively the high-risk patients, on whom more attention should be focused in the future, in an attempt to diminish the frequency of immediate psychiatric complications and to improve the outcome of the operation. Psychotherapeutic interventions should concentrate on certain points.

Research by many groups over the past 20 years has confirmed the hypothesis and demonstrated the complexity of multiple factors at work, (for instance, a combination of pre-operative, operative, and post-operative factors may play a role in delirium). Pre- and post-operative ventilation of feelings seem to contribute to the prevention of delirium, and a pre-operative visit by the nursing staff may help to develop a trusting relationship. Patients should be told pre-operatively that delirium may occur, and should be encouraged to communicate all such symptoms to the staff; they should be reassured that should these occur, it is a common and temporary problem. Patients who are unprepared may fear that they are going crazy or that they have suffered permanent brain damage. While in the recovery room, every effort should be made to reduce sleep interruption and to increase the patient's mobility; family visiting should be encouraged. Following surgery, patients should have an opportunity to review and understand their psychotic experiences and fears, and again, they should be reassured that this is a common occurrence.

An instance of noncompliance which is especially serious and dramatic occurs when a patient leaves the coronary care unit against medical advice (AMA). This disturbing and seemingly self-injurious behavior raises several important questions with regard to the medical and psychological status of these patients. In one study, patients were compared with matched controls on the basis of sociodemographic, medical behavior, and psychiatric variables retrospectively. The AMA group differed significantly from the control group on a number of factors; they were younger, had had a number of previous AMA sign-outs, had less severe medical problems, and gave self-reports of alcoholism and emotional difficulties (Baile et al. 1979).

Needed Areas of Research

In this area, it must be admitted that traditional psychiatric knowledge does not help greatly; teamwork is needed especially by interdisciplinary research groups.

Practical assessment tools are needed to serve as standard assessment instruments for both clinical practice and research; these instruments should be as short as possible and easily mastered to permit use by nonpsychiatrists and nurses; they are needed especially in evaluation of delirium, depression, and anxiety. Attention also has to be paid to the methods which evaluate the patient's quality of life. We need intervention studies to evaluate the effects of information, and to develop support systems and different kinds of psychosocial interventions. Special emphasis should be put on children.

Psychiatrists have to participate in the development of equipment and monitoring techniques – especially noninvasive brain monitoring. Multicenter studies are required so that larger samples can be assessed and different practices compared. Prospective studies are needed so that risk factors can be separated from the consequences of illness or surgery. We also have to be able to identify patients at risk, to whom more attention should be paid.

More knowledge is needed about the culture of patients as well as research on the education of staff; supervisory practices and Balint groups have to be fully evaluated. More knowledge is needed about compliance. Research work also improves collaboration between different medical disciplines: ethical issues should be discussed and a cost/benefit approach emphasized.

Transplantation surgery is a new field, in which the selection and psychological problems of donors need investigation as well as the characteristics of recipients on waiting lists, who seem to have many adjustment problems. Transplantation surgery also has many psychosocial implications for the recipient, the family, and society at large.

Nurses working in research are now providing essential information on themselves, the clients of nursing, and the products and procedures used to effect nursing intervention in clinical settings. The type of information provided by these clinical studies is essential, since nurses, being closest to the patient, are best able to conduct studies which are relevant to patient care and readily applicable to the clinical setting. It is essential that nurses in the clinical area should engage in research, since they have intimate knowledge of patients' problems and of the problems involved in nursing work. Furthermore, nurses are the only personnel who can effectively implement these research findings, particularly in specialized areas of practice, such as perioperative nursing.

References

Baile WF, Brinker JA, Wachspress JD, Engel BT (1979) Signouts against medical advice from a coronary care unit. J Behav Med 2:85–92

Cassem NH, Hacket TP (1971) Psychiatric consultation in a coronary care unit. Ann Intern Med 75:9–14

Crisp AH, Stonehill E (1969) Aspects of the psychological status of patients treated with cardiac pacemakers. Postgrad Med J 45:423

DeNour A, Kaplan H (1976) The psychiatric aspects of renal haemodialysis. In: Howells J (ed) Modern perspectives in the psychiatric aspects of surgery. Brunner/Mazel, New York, pp 343–375

Forester BM, Kornfeld DS, Fleiss J (1978) Psychiatric aspects of radiotherapy. Am J Psychiatry 135:960–963

Gonsalves-Ebrahim L, Sterin G, Dale Gulledge A, Gibson WT, Rodgers DA (1987) Noncompliance in younger adults on hemodialysis. Psychosomatics 28:34–41

Jennet B (1984) High technology medicine: benefits and burdens. Nuffield Provincial Hospital Trust, London

Kimball CP (1977) Psychological responses to the experience of open-heart surgery. In: Moos CH (ed) Coping with physical illness. Plenum, New York, pp 113–133

Kimball CP (ed) (1979) Symposium on liaison psychiatry. The psychiatric clinics of North America, vol 2, no 2. Saunders, Philadelphia

Kornfeld DS (1972) The hospital environment: its impact on the patient. Adv Psychosom Med 8:252–270

Kornfeld DS, Zimberg S, Malm JR (1965) Psychiatric complications of open-heart surgery. N Engl J Med 273:287

Rosch PJ, Kearney HM (1985) Holistic medicine and technology: a modern dialectic. Soc Sci Med 21:1405–1409

Steidl JH, Finkelstein FO, Wexler JP, Feigenbaum H, Kitsen J, Kliger AS, Quinlan DM (1980) Medical condition, adherence to treatment regiments, and family functioning: their interaction in patients receiving long-term dialysis treatment. Arch Gen Psychiatry 37:1025–1027

Tienari P, Outakoski J, Juolasmaa A, Hirvenoja R (1983) Open heart surgery: the psychiatric point of view. In: Krakowski AJ, Kimball CP (eds) Psychosomatic medicine. Plenum New York, pp 113–118

Psychiatric Side-Effects of Nonpsychotropic Drugs

D. Naber and H. Hippius

The detection of adverse drug reactions has long been of interest to both clinicians and researchers. Traditionally, adverse effects have primarily been defined as dysfunctional somatic consequences of drug intake. Nevertheless, investigations of psychotropic drug effects had already started nearly 100 years ago (Kraepelin 1892).

Systematic research on the effects of psychotropic drugs has taken place only during the past decades, parallel to the onset and development of modern psychiatric pharmacotherapy. Investigations on the adverse effects of psychiatric drugs have in fact contributed substantial knowledge, specifically on the behavioral toxicity of psychopharmacotherapeutic treatment. In heightening awareness of the effects of psychotropic drugs, this line of investigation has also fostered interest in the psychotropic effects of nonpsychiatric drugs. Although such effects have occasionally been mentioned in case reports, in clinical trials, and more recently in drug screening programs, comprehensive reports have only just begun to appear (Bullinger 1987; Danielson et al. 1981; D'Arcy 1979; Ellinwood and Petrie 1979; Hall et al. 1980; Hippius and Bullinger 1984; Johnson 1981; Peterson 1980).

Knowledge of the psychotropic effects of nonpsychotropic drugs seems important for three reasons. First, information on adverse effects of psychotropic drugs is essential for efficient and safe pharmacotherapy, i.e., for preventing major psychiatric disturbances as a consequence of drug intake, as well as in helping clinicians to decide at which "cost," in terms of psychological changes, a drug treatment for somatic complaints can or cannot be carried out. Second, knowledge of the psychotropic effects of primarily somatotropic drugs can be useful in generating hypotheses on multifactorial mechanisms of drug action, comprising psychological and physiological components, as well as on their interactions. Thus, research on adverse mental effects of nonpsychiatric drugs can contribute to the identification of psychosomatic relationships underlying drug action in general. Vice versa, it can identify distinct pathways of the transmission and processing of somatopsychic information. Third, and perhaps most important, psychotropic effects, which were originally unwanted or at least unexpected side-effects of somatotropic drugs, could well lead to the de-

Psychiatrische Klinik und Poliklinik der Universität München, Nußbaumstr. 7, D-8000 München 2

Interaction Between Mental and Physical Illness
Edited by R. Öhman et al.

velopment of psychopharmacological agents to treat psychiatric disorders. This was the case with isoniazid, the antitubercular agent. Its side-effects, such as agitation and hypomanic states, stimulated pharmacological research and led to the development of structurally similar drugs, the MAO inhibitors, which are now important in the treatment of depression.

In the psychiatric literature, a psychotropic drug effect is generally defined as one that "alters one or more components of a patient's mood, cognition or gross behavior" (Hall et al. 1980). Such alterations may be therapeutically desired, as in psychopharmacotherapy; may be unexpected, but not necessarily unwanted, as in general medical practice; but may also be considered adverse effects. This usually occurs when a patient's normal functioning is affected by alterations in perceptual and cognitive functions, psychomotor performance, motivation, mood, interpersonal relationships, or intrapsychic processes. While these definitions cover overall impairment of psychological functioning, severe psychiatric symptoms can also be associated with adverse drug effects. Such drug-induced psychotropic effects can be classified in many ways, depending on whether severity, duration, or reversibility of symptoms is considered.

Classification of Psychotropic Effects

The most widely used differentiation of psychotropic effects is that of McClelland (1986) into: (a) behavioral toxicity, (b) delirium, (c) affective reactions, (d) paranoid and schizophrenia-like reactions, (e) hallucinatory states, (f) dementia and pseudodementia, and (g) neuropsychiatric states. Behavioral toxicity refers to changes in activation level (drowsiness vs arousal), disturbances of sleep (sleepiness, insomnia, vivid dreams, nightmares), and a variety of behavioral changes (irritability, anxiety, hostility, changes in sexual behavior). Delirium is the impairment of consciousness manifesting itself in disorientation or hallucination; it is also referred to as a confusional state or acute organic brain syndrome. Affective reactions include depression or mania in mild to severe forms. Depressive symptoms can range from weepiness to depressive psychoses with psychomotor retardation, suicidal ideation, and delusions of guilt; manic symptoms can range from elated mood to overexcitement with aggression or grandiose ideation. Paranoid and schizophrenia-like psychosis is characterized by delusions of persecution in clear consciousness; these psychoses include incoherence of thought and emotional withdrawal. Hallucinatory states usually involve vivid visual hallucinations, but also auditory hallucinations occurring alone or in conjunction with other features of delirium or psychosis. Dementia is the usually irreversible deterioration of intellect, memory, and personality. Neuropsychiatric states refer to various syndromes of mixed neurological or psychiatric symptoms (encephalopathies, movement and speech disorders, extrapyramidal symptoms).

Numerous psychopathological syndromes are included in the above list, and there is probably no single symptom known in psychiatric practice which cannot be induced by drug therapy. Most of the more severe syndromes presenting as psychiatric emergencies are exogenous psychoses. Current literature reveals that three syndromes are observed fairly often: a delirious state in about 50%, a depressive syndrome in about 30%, and a paranoid-hallucinatory syndrome in about 10%. The remaining 10% consists of various other or mixed syndromes. It is well documented that several syndromes can coexist or alternate within one patient. The patient's degree of vigilance is of prognostic importance: If this is disturbed, alterations of affect, delusions, and hallucinations are usually reversible. However, in the case of undisturbed vigilance, the "psychoorganic syndrome" with disorientation, alteration of concentration and memory as well as lability and incontinence of affect is most often at least partly irreversible (Hippius and Bullinger 1984).

Identifying Psychotropic Drug Effects

The process of identifying psychotropic drug effects involves different perceptual and decision-making processes, both from doctors and patients: these mainly involve noticing changes in mood or behavior and attributing these symptoms to a drug (Bullinger 1987). Especially in the case of mild effects, this involves information processing and depends on the patient's sensitivity as well as on the doctor's receptiveness to such symptoms. Problems arise for the doctor when a distinction has to be made between different degrees of psychological change (e.g., lethargy vs depression) and particularly, if the psychiatric symptom could well be related to a somatic disease. For example, after open-heart surgery or other extensive operations, patients often show distinct psychopathological syndromes. The same is true of patients suffering from endocrinopathies and cardiovascular or other severe internal diseases. In these cases, potential psychotropic drug effects are barely detectable.

The process of identifying symptoms as possible drug effects implies the patient's awareness and ability to report changes in his normal mental and emotional state or performance, as well as the medical staff's ability to notice and report a change in the patient's mood, cognitive function, or behavior. In the case of the patient, this process not only involves awareness and interpretation of changes, but also readiness to report symptoms, which is dependent on the patient-doctor relationship and on compliance. In general, a patient's reaction to a drug is embedded in a variety of nonpharmacological factors, and this has been demonstrated in studies of adverse nondrug reactions, which reveal a closer association between adverse effects and personality characteristics than between adverse effects and drugs (Bulpitt and Dollery 1979; Silverman 1979). In the case of the doctor, noticing psychopathological changes depends both on his knowledge of the patient and on his alertness to such changes.

Having noticed a change in the patient's mood, cognitive function, or behavior, the second step is the attribution of this psychopathological symptom to a drug. For the doctor, this involves gathering information on the phenomenology of mental changes, on the modes of drug intake, on drug metabolism, as well as on factors affecting drug effects, such as interactions with other drugs and the incidence of adverse mental effects with a particular drug, based on clinical experience or literature reports. When symptoms appear that have not previously been related to the drug, the discovery of a relationship between a drug and psychopathological change is a matter of serendipity for the professional staff.

Generally speaking, psychological or psychiatric symptoms can be attributed to drug action if they occur shortly after the intake of a drug, stop after its discontinuation, correlate with biochemical levels of the substance in blood, urine, or CSF, do not fit the clinical picture for which the drug was given, and occur again with reexposure to the drug. Attributing a symptom to a drug, however, does not depend only on information as such, but also on how it is used to form a diagnostically or therapeutically relevant judgement: there usually is "known data, but unknown human data processing" (Hogarth 1980). For example, interobserver variability, even between experts, is considerable. In a report of 500 suspected adverse drug reactions, evaluated by clinical pharmacologists, only 21% were definitely diagnosed as such, while in the remaining 79%, there was disagreement on the causal agent (Koch-Weser et al. 1977). Recent investigations have specifically examined the processes by which a doctor arrives at attributing symptoms to drugs. There are four major factors jeopardizing the correct detection of adverse effects (Hammond and Joyce 1977):

1. Compliance: drug effects may occur at lower dosage than reported or may be due to other drugs than those reported
2. Illusionary associations: misattribution because of distorted event perception
3. Modes of judgement ranging from the analytical-experimental to the intuitive, which result in inexplicit individual bases for judgement
4. Range of effects in using different rating scales to judge drug responses

Other factors include observer fatigue and the recency or saliency of data features. To tackle the problem of unknown data processing, the use of decision algorithms has been proposed: these are formalized procedures to identify single adverse drug reactions. Hutchinson et al. (1983) have suggested a detailed algorithmic method, which involves: (a) previous general experience with the drug, (b) excluding alternative etiological candidates, (c) timing of events, (d) recording drug levels and evidence of overdose, (e) dechallenge, and (f) rechallenge. Using this method, the authors obtained a 66% agreement in 80 suspected adverse drug reactions.

As discussed above, detection and attribution of adverse effects is highly dependent on the subjective appraisals and judgements of both patients and clinicians. Therefore, and for other methodological reasons, reports of adverse drug effects may not be unequivocal. In general, reports on adverse effects are derived from three sources: (a) spontaneous reporting (e.g., letters to journal editors), (b) case-control studies (retrospective and prospective clinical trials), and (c) cohort and epidemiological studies.

These sources have various advantages and disadvantages. While spontaneous reports are useful in transmitting new information, they do not provide enough evidence to generalize from the cases reported and sometimes represent false-positive findings. Case control studies, if carried out correctly, are valuable in this respect, but rarely include systematic documentation of adverse mental effects. Retrospective cohort studies comprise many patients, but do not allow the inclusion of potentially influential factors. Prospective studies are unlikely to comprise new information because of a delay between first reports of adverse reactions and their inclusion in the screening program (Griffin and D'Arcy 1981). Therefore, and because of the problems in the identification of adverse drug reactions, information on the psychotropic effects of nonpsychotropic drugs should be very critically evaluated.

Pathomechanism of Psychotropic Effects

The pathomechanisms or etiology of a psychotropic effect also need to be very critically evaluated. There is now abundant evidence that the same drug induces very different psychopathological syndromes in different patients, and that even within one patient, drug-induced symptoms can change in an unpredictable way (Hippius and Bullinger 1984). The nonspecific relationship between drug and psychotropic effect is caused by a multitude of factors which influence the psychological outcome of drug intake (see Fig. 1).

These factors are related to the drug, disease, individual disposition, and social situation. With regard to the drug, dosage and duration of therapy, pharmacokinetics, mode of intake, and other factors have to be considered, e.g., how fast was the dosage increased or decreased. Disease-related factors include the kind of illness and stage or severity, influencing the drug's effect. Individual-specific factors are variables such as age, sex, somatic and psychiatric history, family history, knowledge about medicine in general and the drug in particular, personality variables, coping styles, etc. Social factors such as the patient-doctor relationship, and inpatient vs outpatient status also seem to be important. All these factors influence the way in which a drug affects CNS structures. Drugs acting directly on the CNS are more likely to produce psychiatric side-effects than those administered to control peripheral organs and systems. However, some of the latter drugs can cross the blood-brain barrier, and thus also exert a CNS effect. The action of the drug on the CNS may also be mediated by psychological processes, especially with regard to the milder symptoms. In fact, it seems tempting to speculate that in the absence of direct physiological CNS effects, a drug may subjectively be judged psychotropic and then lead to secondary CNS activation, producing the psychotropic effect.

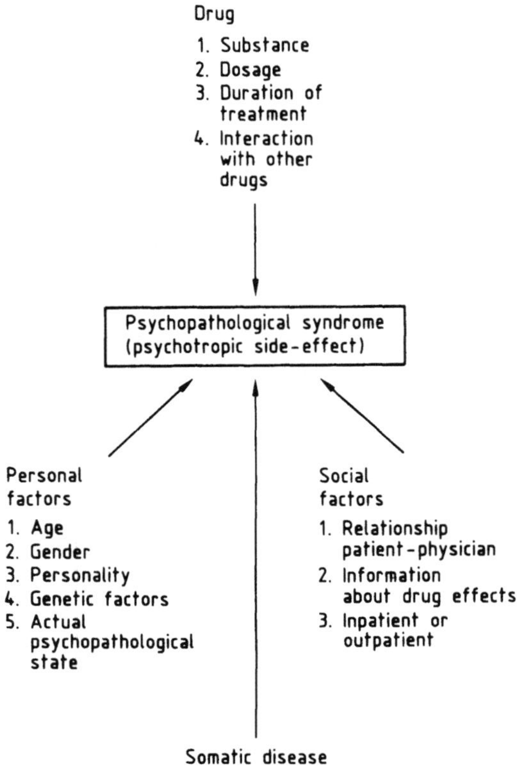

Fig. 1. Multifactorial etiology of psychotropic effects

Adverse placebo effects are usually somatic alterations like sickness, vomiting, headache, dry mouth, and agitation. However, psychotropic placebo effects are also quite common and range from mild symptoms such as alterations of concentration and memory, fatigue, or depression, to impressive symptoms like confusion and dependence. The underlying psychological mechanisms are barely known, but research on placebo suggests that personality characteristics, situational factors, and cognitive sets determine the therapeutic efficacy of drugs as well as the adverse effects experienced with drug intake (Silverman 1979).

Psychotropic Effects of the Different Nonpsychotropic Drugs

The line between psychotropic and nonpsychotropic drugs is hard to draw. Nearly each drug has, at least in the subtoxic range, some psychotropic effects. Therefore, drugs which are not primarily used to treat psychiatric syndromes are considered to be nonpsychotropic and are included in the following short review (see Table 1).

Table 1. Psychotropic effects of nonpsychotropic drugs (from Bullinger 1987)

	Behavioral toxicity	Delirium	Affective reactions	Paranoid schizophrenia-like reactions	Hallucinatory states	Dementia	Neuropsychiatric states
Aminophylline	+	+			+		
Amphetamines	+		+	+	?		
Analgesics	+	+	+		+		
Antihistamines	+	+		+			
Anticonvulsants		+	+				
Clonidine			+				
Methyldopa	+		+				
Propanolol			?	?		+	
Reserpine			+				+
Anticholinergics	+	+					
Chloroquine		+					
Corticosteroids	+	+	+	+			
Digitalis glycosides	+	+	+		+		
Oral contraceptives	+		+				
Amantadine	+	+				+	
L-Dopa	+	+	+	+	+	+	+
Tuberculostatics	+	+				+	
Procainpenicilline		+					
Sulfonamides			+		+		
Opiates					+		

Central Nervous System Stimulants

Amphetamines are used therapeutically for the treatment of narcolepsy and hyperactivity or as anorectic agents; they are often abused for their activating effects. It has been known for a long time that their use, and specifically abuse, provokes psychoses in both nonpsychiatric and psychiatric populations (Janowsky and Risch 1979). Since the psychotic syndrome is often indistinguishable from paranoid schizophrenia, amphetamine psychoses have been extensively investigated as pharmacological models for schizophrenia. Single doses of therapeutic range usually induce euphoria and a sense of heightened perception, but occasionally also compulsive behavior, depression, delusions, and hallucinations. The variation in individual responses is particularly large in hyperactive children with minimal brain dysfunction who are receiving methylphenidate (Cowart 1982).

Within the group of sympathomimetic drugs, phenylephedrine, a nasal decongestant, has been reported to have the potential of psychic dependence, in terms of a ritual use, and to be associated with toxic psychosis. For instance, a 26-year-old woman without previous psychiatric history who had taken phenylephedrine every 15 min for 13 days, developed hallucinations and delusions (Snow et al. 1980). Pseudoephedrine has also been related to anxiety and to toxic psychosis (Lopatin et al. 1981). In children up to 15 years of age, symptoms ranged from restlessness, irritation, aggressiveness and sleep disturbances, to severe psychotic disorders, which included confusion, visual hallucinations, vivid paranoid misconceptions, and acute maniform psychoses (Diaz et al. 1979).

The most prominent adverse effects of anorectic drugs or appetite suppressants include insomnia and nervousness, but other symptoms, similar to those from amphetamine, have also been reported (Douglas and Munro 1982).

Aminophylline and related compounds, used chiefly in the treatment of asthma, have also been reported to induce dizziness, anxiety, agitation, insomnia, depression, and psychosis (Lamont et al. 1979; Murphy et al. 1981).

Analgesics

Analgesics can induce psychiatric symptoms through acute intoxication, long-term administration (sometimes in a therapeutic dosage), and after withdrawal. Most prominent are the psychotropic effects of opiates, in particular of pentazocine: this drug is often abused, alone or in combination with other drugs, for its psychoactive effects and is likely to produce a variety of neuropsychiatric symptoms, including depression, anxiety, fatigue, irritation, and decreased libido. Of patients receiving pentazocine, 2%–8% develop hallucinations and bizarre feelings within 10 days of treatment (Danielson et al. 1981). Rebound effects have also been reported during withdrawal from pentazocine. These psychotic symptoms are interesting in relation to the endorphin hypothesis for schizophrenia.

Not only opiates, but also other analgesics can lead to dependency, abuse, and a variety of psychiatric symptoms. Acetylsalicylic acid, for example, is known to produce a wide range of symptoms from psychomotor agitation and irritability to impairment of consciousness. In two children, acetylsalicylic acid treatment reportedly led to confusion, loss of consciousness, and convulsions (Makela et al. 1980). Dementia has also been found to be a rare consequence of acetylsalicylic acid abuse (Murray et al. 1979).

About 30% of patients taking phenacetin-containing analgesics suffer from symptoms such as irritability, depression and, less often, hallucinations (Del Favero 1981). The effects of indomethacin are similar: disturbed concentration, depression with suicidal behavior at times, and hallucinations occur. However, a recent study investigating indomethacin versus other medication in 461 patients did not find that any psychiatric effects were mentioned (Boussina et al. 1983). In normal volunteers, a single dose of 75 mg indomethacin also produced only minimal central side-effects such as dizziness (Duesing et al. 1983). Nevertheless, in contrast to these trials, single case studies continue to report psychiatric symptomatology associated with indomethacin.

Cardiovascular Drugs

Psychiatric symptoms such as psychosis, depression, and delirium following cardiovascular drug treatment have very often been reported. Within the group of cardiac glycosides, digitalis intoxication has received special attention because of its CNS effects, which include restlessness and agitation. Digitalis intoxication is involved in transient global amnesia, in anxiety psychoses with visual and auditory hallucinations, and in paranoid delusions in clear consciousness. A constellation of symptoms, often referred to as "digitalis delirium," has been observed repeatedly and is characterized by incoherent thinking, disturbed orientation, difficulty in comprehension, illusions, hallucinations, delusional thought, irritability, distractability and labile mood. Digitalis delirium reportedly has a higher incidence in elderly patients (Danielson et al. 1981; Singh et al. 1977).

Quinidine, and other drugs used to treat arrhythmias, have been associated with delirious states, but the symptoms are reported to remit promptly on discontinuation of the drug (Lloyd and Greenblatt 1981). Diuretics also have been associated with psychological effects, which do not directly involve the CNS, but rather seem to be due to electrolyte imbalance. The potassium depleting action of diuretics, with a subsequent hypokalemic state, has been related to a wide range of symptoms, ranging from apathy to depression, confusion, and hallucinations (Paykel et al. 1982).

Minor neuropsychiatric symptoms such as light-headedness, insomnia, fatigue, but also visual hallucinations have been causally related to long-term treatment with β-blockers (Laake 1981). In a recent study, 84 women, who were all approximately 50 years old, were treated with β-blockers and reported side-effects such as sleep disturbances (34%), nightmares (13%), a general feeling of tiredness (40%), melancholy and depression (40%). But a comparison of these patients with a control group showed no statistically significant difference in the incidence of side-effects between the groups, suggesting that such minor psychic complaints are common in this type of population and that no specific adverse effects of β-blockers could be identified (Bengtsson et al. 1980).

More severe psychiatric symptoms have also been reported during treatment with propanolol. Psychoses with visual hallucinations, disorientation, and confusion are likely to begin at the commencement of therapy, as well as after long-term use with increasing doses. Thus drug-induced psychosis is not bound to clinical populations, but can also be provoked in healthy normal volunteers (Horn et al. 1982; White and Riotte 1982).

Side-effects of hypotensive drugs have been investigated extensively, with particular attention to these drugs' potential for inducing depression. The mechanisms of effect appear to be either central action, cholinergic blockade, adrenergic blockade, or modification of the effector response. Among the centrally acting drugs, methyldopa and clonidine have been found to cause sedation in almost all cases, depression in 2%–4%, and sleep disorders in 2%–5%

of patients. Various other reported effects include impaired concentration, anxiety, paranoia, hallucinations, and confusional states, the latter especially occurring in psychiatrically vulnerable cases (Kulkarni et al. 1984). Depending on the mental symptom present, the mechanism of the psychotic effect is believed to be either hypoadrenergic (depression with clonidine administration) or hyperadrenergic (mania on clonidine withdrawal). The observations, however, that withdrawal can also be associated with schizophrenia-like symptoms and that clonidine also has anticonvulsant properties imply more complex mechanisms.

Anticonvulsants

Adverse psychiatric effects of anticonvulsants mostly involve a slowing of mental processes, but hallucinations and affective responses have also been observed (Diehl 1983). The effects of phenytoin, primidone, and valproate most frequently are produced by overdose and intoxication and since psychopathology correlates well with drug plasma levels, most psychiatric effects can be predicted and avoided.

Studies on the cognitive effects of anticonvulsant medication indicate a beneficial effect from reduction of polypharmacy, as well as from a change to carbamazepine. Patients who were already on carbamazepine had the best test results, suggesting a positive effect of carbamazepine on performance and mood (Thompson and Trimble 1982).

Drugs for Parkinson's Disease

Drugs for the treatment of Parkinson's disease, such as biperiden, due to their anticholinergic properties, induce sedation and drowsiness up to toxic confusional states. However, in some individuals and in particular in neuroleptic-treated patients, they also have stimulant effects and cause euphoria, agitation, and hallucinations. That is probably why schizophrenic patients often abuse these drugs (Jellinek 1977).

L-Dopa therapy induces a variety of psychiatric symptoms including sleep disturbances (20%), depression (9%), confusion (13%), and hallucinations (2%). Psychotic symptoms appear to be more common when enzyme inhibitors or anticholinergic drugs are also used (Leibner 1977; Moskowitz et al. 1978). Bromocriptine has similar psychotropic effects – up to 10% of cases may have to be withdrawn from treatment because of confusion, hallucinations, and delusions (Einarson 1983). These dopamine-related effects give strong support to the dopamine-hypothesis for schizophrenia.

Steroids

Over the past 30 years, many psychiatric side-effects of corticosteroid therapy have been reported (Carpenter and Gruen 1982). In 1972, the incidence of prednisone-associated mental disturbances was reported to be 3% of all treated patients (Boston Collaborative Drug Surveillance Program 1972): the most prominent adverse mental effects are affective disorders with manic or depressive syndromes, as well as psychoses with paranoid and hallucinatory syndromes (Ling et al. 1981). However, information on this subject is still sparse, and derived mostly from older studies. For example, in 550 corticosteroid-treated patients, compared with an equal-sized control group, the incidence of psychosis was 3.2% in the untreated and 1.8% in the treated group (Smyllie and Conolly 1968).

Another study, however, found that acute psychosis developed in 12% of a sample of 50 treated patients, whereas in a control sample, the incidence of psychosis was only 2.6% (Marx and Barker 1967). While earlier work suggested that neither dosage nor duration of treatment affects time of onset, duration, type or severity of disturbance, corticosteroid psychoses were recently reported to occur within the first 6 days of treatment, the severity of the symptoms being dose-related (Hall et al. 1979). A review of 55 anecdotal cases revealed that 31% of the cases involved hypomania, 40% involved depression, and 11% were diagnosed as bipolar illness. In 16%, acute psychotic reactions, characterized by delusions, hallucinations, stupor, and catatonia were found, and one patient described experiencing anxiety and agitation during corticosteroid treatment (Ling et al. 1981). It should be noted that in 23% of these anecdotal cases, patients had previously experienced psychiatric symptoms, suggesting that mental disturbances during medication might reflect the premorbid pattern of personality. In this context, the well-documented elevated cortisol levels in serum and CSF of depressed patients are of considerable interest.

Oral Contraceptives

Since the introduction of hormonal contraceptives, mood changes, sexual disturbances, psychovegetative symptoms, phobic anxiety, and psychotic reactions have been reported. The problem of attributing such symptoms to oral contraceptive intake, however, is complicated by intervening psychological factors in terms of personality, drug appraisal (Dennerstein and Burrows 1979), and by interactions of oral contraceptives with other drugs (Beckenridge et al. 1979). In an earlier double-blind study involving 400 women, no significant difference in the frequency of depression or loss of libido could be demonstrated as a consequence of contraceptive intake, compared with placebo (Goldzieher et al. 1971). In a general practitioner survey, carried out on 686 women, the incidence of depression among the 335 users was not higher than among matched controls, even though there was a correlation between depression and neuroticism scores in users. In addition, the intensity of depression appeared to be related to socioeconomic factors and personality rather than to contraceptive intake (Fleming and Seagar 1978). A review by Slap (1981) reported that in 9 out of 12 clinical studies, oral contraceptives were believed to have caused depression in 16%–56% of patients; in the remaining three studies no association of this kind was observed. These mood changes appear to depend on the relative proportions of estrogen and progestogen in the contraceptive formulation as well as the patient's previous history of emotional lability (Glick and Bennett 1981).

Therapeutic administration of female sex hormones for menopausal disorders can also have psychotropic effects. Mood improvements with estrogen have been confirmed, effects of estradiol and progestogen on mood in postmenopausal women were also investigated (DeLignières and Vincens 1982): The relationship between mood and plasma levels included a correlation between low pre- and posttreatment estradiol plasma levels and moderate depression and between higher estradiol levels and increased well-being. Excessive increase, however, was associated with unpleasant effects, such as irritability and aggressiveness. Thus, the potential beneficial effects of sex hormones on mood seem to be dose-dependent, and care should be taken to adjust the dose appropriately for individual patients.

Conclusions

A variety of psychological and psychiatric disturbances are reportedly suspected reactions to a large number of drugs but, although these reports have made doctors aware of the possibility of such reactions, they have not firmly established a causal relationship in all cases.

This is because published evidence has come from sources with differences in diagnostic criteria, in methods of assessment and validation of suspected reactions, and in the degree of attention given to such predisposing factors as drug intolerance, concurrent physical disease, and preexisting mental instability. Necessary to improve the situation is greater awareness of the multiple factors involved in the production of adverse reactions, better ways of assessing these factors, and a standardized method of detecting and categorizing mental changes suspected of being caused by drug therapy.

The hope that the study of adverse reactions will provide clues to the biochemical mechanisms responsible for some idiopathic mental disorders has not been fulfilled yet, though there have been some developments in this direction.

References

Beckenridge AM, Back DJ, Orme M (1979) Interactions between oral contraceptives and other drugs. Pharmacol Ther 7:617–622

Bengtsson C, Lennartsson J, Lindquist O, Noppa H, Sigurdsson J (1980) Sleep disturbances, nightmares and other possible central nervous disturbances in a population sample of women, with special reference to those on antihypertensive drugs. J Clin Pharmacol 17:173–182

Boston Collaborative Drug Surveillance Program (1972) Acute adverse reactions to prednisone in relation to dosage. Clin Pharmacol Ther 13:694–719

Boussina I, Guenther W, Marti Masso R (1983) Double-blind multicenter study comparing meclofenamate sodium with indomethacin and placebo in the treatment of extraarticular rheumatic disease. Arzneimittelforschung 33:649–653

Bullinger M (1987) Psychotropic effects of non-psychotropic drugs. Adv Drug React Ac Pois Rev 3:141–167

Bulpitt CJ, Dollery CT (1979) Evaluation of the symptoms of treated hypertensive patients. Methods Inf Med 18:36–44

Carpenter WT, Gruen PH (1982) Cortisol's effect on human mental functioning. J Clin Psychopharmacol 2:91–98

Cowart VS (1982) Stimulant therapy for attention disorders. JAMA 248:279–782

Danielson DA, Porter JB, Lawson DH, Soubrie C, Jick H (1981) Drug-associated psychiatric disturbances in medical inpatients. Psychopharmacology (Berlin) 74:105–111

D'Arcy PF (1979) Drug-induced psychiatric disorders. In: D'Arcy PF, Griffin JP (eds) Iatrogenic diseases, 2nd edn. Oxford University Press, London, pp 324–340

Del Favero A (1981) Anti-inflammatory analgesics and drugs used in rheumatism and gout. In: Dukes MNG (ed) Side effects of drugs, annual 5. Excerpta Medica, Amsterdam, pp 88–118

DeLignières M, Vincens M (1982) Differential effects of exogenous oestradiol and progesterone on mood in post-menopausal women: individual dose-effect relationship. Maturitas 4:67–74

Dennerstein L, Burrows GD (1979) Affect and the menstrual cycle. J Affective Disord 1:77–83

Diaz MA, Wise T, Semchyshyn G (1979) Self-medication with pseudoephredine in a chronically depressed patient. Am J Psychiatry 136:1217–1220

Diehl LW (1983) Psychotrope Effekte der Antiepilektika. Psychiatr Clin 16:305–310

Douglas JG, Munro JF (1982) Drug treatment and obesity. Pharmacol Ther 18:351–356

Duesing R, Dittrich P, Kukovetz WR, Lehmann K, Kramer HJ (1983) Indomethacin kinetics and urinary excretion of prostaglandin E2 following oral administration of various dosage forms of indomethacin. Z Rheumatol 42:235–242

Einarson TR (1983) Psychotic reactions to low-dose bromocriptine. Clin Pharm 2:273–276

Ellinwood EH, Petric WM (1979) Drug-induced psychoses. In: Pickens R, Heston L (eds) Psychiatric factors in drug abuse. Grune and Stratton, New York, pp 301–337

Fleming O, Seagar CP (1978) Incidence of depressive symptoms in users of the oral contraceptive. Psychiatry 132:431–437

Glick ID, Bennett MD (1981) Psychiatric complications of progesterone and oral contraceptives. J Clin Psychopharmacol 1:350–361

Goldzieher JW, Moses E, Averkin E, Scheel C, Taber B (1971) Nervousness and depression attributed to oral contraceptives. A double blind, placebo-controlled study. Am J Obstet Gynecol 111:1013–1019

Griffin JP, D'Arcy PF (1981) Adverse reactions to drugs – the information lag. In: Dukes MNG (ed) Side effects of drugs, annual 5. Excerpta Medica, Amsterdam, pp 15–24

Hall RCW, Popkin MK, Stickney SK, Gardener ER (1979) Presentation of the "steroid" psychosis. J Nerv Ment Dis 167:229–236

Hall RCW, Stickney SK, Gardener ER (1980) Behavioral toxicity of non-psychiatric drugs. In: Hall RCW (ed) Psychiatric presentations of medical illness: somatopsychic disorders. MTP, New York, pp 337–349
Hammond KR, Joyce CRB (1977) Psychological influences on human judgement, especially of adverse effects. In: Gross FH, Inman WH (eds) Drug monitoring. Academic, London, pp 269–287
Hippius H, Bullinger M (1984) Psychische Störungen. In: Rahn KH (ed) Erkrankungen durch Arzneimittel. Thieme, Stuttgart, pp 544–560
Hogarth RM (1980) Judgement, drug monitoring and decision aids. In: Inman WHW (ed) Monitoring for drug safety. MTP, Lancaster, pp 439–475
Horn JR, Rylander ML, Hicks HM (1982) Propanolol induced hallucinosis. Clin Pharm 1:464–472
Hutchinson TA, Flegel KM, Ho Pingkong H, Bloom WS, Kramer MS, Trummer EG (1983) Reasons for disagreement in the standardized assessment of suspected adverse drug reactions. Clin Pharmacol Ther 34:421–429
Janowsky DS, Risch C (1979) Amphetamine psychosis and psychotic symptoms. Psychopharmacology 65:73–79
Jellinek TC (1977) Mood elevating effects of trihexyphenidyl and biperiden in individuals taking antipsychotic medication. Dis Nerv Syst 38:353–357
Johnson DAW (1981) Drug-induced psychiatric disorders. Drugs 22:53–60
Koch-Weser J, Sellers CM, Zacest R (1977) The ambiguity of adverse drug reactions. Eur J Clin Pharmacol 11:75–82
Kraepelin E (1892) Über die Beeinflussung einfacher psychischer Vorgänge durch einige Arzneimittel. Experimentelle Untersuchungen. Fischer, Jena
Kulkarni SK, Mehta AK, Kunchandy J (1984) Some noncardiovascular actions of clonidine. Drugs Today 20:497–509
Laake K (1981) Antianginal and beta-adrenoceptor blocking drugs. In: Dukes MNG (ed) Side effects of drugs, annual 5. Excerpta Medica, Amsterdam, pp 184–204
Lamont H, Van der Straeten M, Meerman E, Bogaert M, Pauwels H (1979) Clinical study of a sustained-release theophylline preparation in asthmatic adults. Curr Med Res Opin 6:132–140
Leibner L (1977) Psychological side effects of L-dopa and anticonvulsant medication. NY State J Med 77:1098–1103
Ling MHM, Perry PJ, Tsuang MT (1981) Side effects of corticosteroid therapy: psychiatric effects. Arch Gen Psychiatry 38:471–475
Lloyd BL, Greenblatt DJ (1981) Neuropsychiatric sequelac of pharmacotherapy of cardiac arrythmias and hypertension. J Clin Psychopharmacol 1:394–401
Lopatin AS, Lavretsky IG, Astahova AV (1981) Central nervous system stimulants and anorectic agents. In: Dukes MNG (ed) Side effects of drugs, annual 5. Excerpta Medica, Amsterdam, pp 1–15
Makela AL, Lang H, Korpela P (1980) Toxic encephalopathy with hyperammonaemia during high dose salicylate therapy. Acta Neurol Scand 61:146–149
Marx FW, Barker WF (1967) Surgical results in patients with ulcerative colitis treated with and without corticosteroids. Am J Surg 113:157–166
McClelland HA (1986) Psychiatric disorders. In: Davies DM (ed) Textbook of adverse drug reactions. Oxford University Press, Oxford, pp 549–577
Moskowitz C, Moses H, Klawans H (1978) Levodopa induced psychosis: a kinding phenomenon. Am J Psychiatry 135:669–674
Murphy B, Dillon A, Fitzgerald M (1981) Theophylline and depression. Br Med J 281:1322
Murray RM, Greene JG, Adams JH (1979) Analgesic abuse and dementia. Lancet II:242
Paykel ES, Fleminger R, Watson JP (1982) Psychiatric side effects of antihypertensive drugs other than reserpine. J Clin Psychopharmacol 2:14–21
Peterson GC (1980) Organic mental disorders induced by drugs or poisons. In: Freedman AM, Kaplan HI (eds) Comprehensive textbook of psychiatry, 3rd edn. Williams and Wilkins, Baltimore, pp 1437–1451

Silverman G (1979) Placebo effect and changes in response set with re-testing: a further source of bias. Neuropharmacology 18:1019–1027
Singh RB, Gupta OR, Gupta HM (1977) Psychosis: a rare manifestation of digoxin intoxication. J Indian Med Assoc 69:62–70
Slap G (1981) Oral contraceptives and depression. J Adolesc Health Care 2:53–61
Smyllie HC, Connolly CK (1968) Incidence of serious complications of corticosteroid therapy in respiratory disease. Thorax 23:571–579
Snow SS, Logan TP, Hollender MH (1980) Nasal spray "addiction" and psychosis: a case report. Br J Psychiatry 136:297–300
Thompson PJ, Trimble MR (1982) Anticonvulsant drugs and cognitive functions. Epilepsia 23:531–542
White WB, Riotte K (1982) Propanolol and white rabbits. N Engl J Med 307:559–563

Psychological Contributions to the Causes and Course of Physical Illness

R. C. B. AITKEN

Introduction

The psychological contributions to the causes and course of physical illness is a topic susceptible to misunderstanding. In the first place, the word psychosomatic should refer to the interrelationship of psychological and medical aspects of any disease or injury. It can be used to reflect a bio-psycho-social approach to diagnosis and treatment, with an assurance that factors in all three dimensions are being taken into account. There should be as much interest in the aetiology of distress as of disease.

The publication of the International Classification of Impairments, Disabilities and Handicaps (WHO 1980) was important because of the distinction denoted by these terms, perhaps more easily remembered as "disease, disablement and disadvantage". Disability refers to reduced function while handicap is the subsequent social disadvantage. Therapy is prescribed in order to minimise disability, while clinical management implies a wider responsibility to reduce social disadvantage. Psychological factors can influence the amount of disturbance in any aspect, and so may require attention at any level (Aitken 1984).

It is recognised that the relationship of the therapist with the patient and his family can be a crucial component in establishing a diagnosis and in the effectiveness of treatment. It is accepted that any carer, not solely the doctor, can influence outcome and so the psychosomatic approach should be adopted by all carers, whether professionals or relatives. The less effective the treatment for any disease or injury, the more important become the psychosocial aspects. Outcome in psychosocial terms is often as much determined by features in the patient as a person as in the disease from which he suffers. In other words, patients with similar diseases and disabilities may have a wide range of handicap. Features of dependency and of motivation are important in determining the outcome of rehabilitation for disability. Both these concepts would benefit from more study in a clinical context.

Rehabilitation Studies Unit, University of Edinburgh, Princess Margaret Rose Hospital, Fairmilehead, Edinburgh EH10 7ED, Scotland, UK

Interaction Between Mental and Physical Illness
Edited by R. Öhman et al.

Theoretical Concepts

Presentation of theory followed by practical action can do much to advance knowledge. For instance, biological consideration of functional psychoses led to advances in psychopharmacology, which in turn stimulated developments of rating scales and improved classification. Psychosomatic conditions would benefit now from the stimulus of a new theory.

The concept of identification of personality type in certain "psychosomatic" diseases, or the theory of specificity, was based on false evidence. The patients studied by psychoanalysis were not representative of those with a disease, and little is likely to be gained by further examination of that theory. There is still interest in behaviour type, certainly with respect to coronary artery disease, but despite much endeavour little certain knowledge has been gained, and so far nothing that has led to much ameliorative action (Johnston 1985).

The concept of alexithymia was similarly based on weak experimental evidence in that the patients studied were mainly those referred for psychotherapy. The concept does not have a strong association with any disease in wider samples of patients. It was a useful stimulus to enquiry at an individual level, when interest was flagging in the theory of specificity.

Research on the effects of stressful life-events has been a useful stimulus in epidemiology. The methodology is treacherous, with many flaws in past studies, but the topic still seems worth pursuing (Creed 1985). Sophisticated methods are necessary and their use may have to be confined to only a few academic centres.

Psycho-physiological changes in connection with stress-coping mechanisms have been demonstrated as factors influencing many symptoms, such as hyperventilation or gastric acidity. The evidence remains unproven for their role in aetiology of pathology, though the progress of certain diseases like breast cancer appears to be influenced by them (Greer et al. 1979). Their relationship with other causes, such as those involving the immune system, seems worthy of more attention (Baker 1987). What makes patients adopt sick role behaviour is also very important, e.g. when coping with the stress of a life-threatening, painful, or chronic disease.

A new theory would be welcome, and it would be valuable to have a proposal in the realm of symptom perception, patient/doctor behaviour, cultural expectations, and communication. This theory would require to take account of sociological as much as psychological concepts. It should generate hypotheses for why people behave in certain ways in response to an awareness of feelings which are judged to be abnormal.

There is an urgent need for a new nomenclature about psychosomatic matters. No present system of classification is adequate to take account of various aspects of psychological disturbance in physical disease or of physical symptoms associated with psychiatric disorder (Lloyd 1986).

Clinical syndromes should be described in multi-axial dimensions; for instance, it is appropriate to classify separately impairment, disability, and handicap, since one cannot be deduced from the other. Likewise independent ratings are required in biological, psychological, and social dimensions. Classifications need to be problem-orientated. Pre-morbid personality and emotional/cognitive reaction should be assessed for inclusion in a universal classification for every patient with serious chronic disease. Knowledge of social adaptation in its several dimensions needs to be recorded.

Methods of measurement need to be reviewed continually and improved for two purposes which are separate – for research, using academic staff, and for clinical practice, using clinical staff; the latter will not readily use sophisticated methods nor be willing to devote much time to the requirements, since clinical methods need to be simple and produce results quickly in meaningful terms (Aitken 1969). Some schedules and rating scales need to have more universal appeal and should not be prepared for a particular study. For this, much could be gained by international acceptance of a method like the Present State Examination has been accepted for schizophrenia. A new classification needs to take account of "psychosomatic" symptoms and psychosocial behaviour.

The Edinburgh Rehabilitation Status Scale (ERSS; Affleck et al. 1988) measures four dimensions in which changes may occur in the course of a disabling illness or during rehabilitation: independence, activity, social integration, and effects of symptoms on lifestyle. It provides a profile of measures, the scores of which can be summated to indicate the overall level of performance of individuals or groups; it can be used either by individual professional staff or by a multiprofessional team. Because ERSS is not tied to any special theoretical assumptions, its data can serve as outcome-dependent variables in any type of research study, as well as for measuring staff workloads and other costs involved in the management of disabled patients.

For the psychosomatic patient, the classification needs to be action-orientated, able to identify "process" and "dynamic analysis" rather than simply categorise. Levels of functioning such as in coping with disability need to be recorded. Separation within a classification such as of a diagnosis is only useful when there are implications for treatment or another aspect of clinical management.

Relevant Known Causes of Disease

The evidence is beyond any doubt that behaviours such as smoking nicotine, drinking alcohol, and taking other drugs are important causes of serious disease. Behaviour relating to exercise, diet, promiscuous sex, and irresponsible vehicle driving is also relevant. To change these behaviours, when they are abnormal, has proved to be one of the greatest challenges facing health educationists. The evidence for their importance has been beyond doubt for many years, and yet it has so far proved extremely difficult to change attitudes and improve behaviour though there are some recent signs for hope. Even when an important factor on alcohol consumption like cost has been identified, governments have been reluctant to increase taxes for beneficial purposes.

The psychological aspects of health education deserve much more study. Communication is a complicated topic, with its problems now better identified and its features researched, such as for marketing purposes and concerning the role of the media. Research to help eradicate smoking and to reduce alcohol consumption should be given higher priority. For instance, there are too few active academic departments working on drinking or smoking studies. More research is required on the basic psychological effects of both nicotine and alcohol; just as it is required on the basic factors affecting response to communication about health in both emotional and behavioural terms. What factors influence attitude changes in the population toward behaviour modification?

Greater attention should be given to psychological aspects of known causes of diseases, rather than to speculative ones like personality influence, except as a dependent variable. A priority should be the study of factors opposing application of what is already known to be beneficial, such as in health education.

Brain Damage

Brain damage after either head injury or stroke requires greater attention with regard to younger patients. The acute services have improved considerably and are generally considered acceptable, but later services for chronic morbidity are still much less effective for a variety of important problems (Meier et al. 1987).

As yet, there is no standardised, sensitive, clinical assessment for neurological disability. It would be valuable to have simple screening tests for cognitive and emotional dysfunction that can be widely used. Increased understanding about the influence of premorbid personality and of the effects of the brain damage on inter-personal relationships would also be valuable. The use of microcomputers for the re-acquisition of skills for perceptual abnormality should have considerable potential. Available measures with increased sensitivity to detect the effects on brain function of other disorders, like that associated with coronary artery bypass surgery, are still needed (Mayou 1986). The simple screening of cognitive impairment is important to detect minor brain damage. It might then encourage prevention or reveal the reduced potential to improve function and to relearn social skills, such as in multiple sclerosis (Ron 1986) or degenerative vascular disease. For too long such damage seems to go unrecognised.

Many severely brain-damaged patients are cared for by their families at home, with professional care only for a limited time. The carers' preceptions of the brain-damaged patient's problems, and the effect of these on their own mental health need further study, including the value of preventive measures.

There has been an increase in knowledge of the subtle effects of brain damage on behaviour and emotion, which have been shown to be very disturbing for both patients and their relatives over a prolonged period.

Psychosomatic Aspects of Known High-Risk Groups

Social Disadvantages

The health implications for people thought likely to have a higher incidence of either psychological or physical morbidity and even mortality require continuing study. Lower socio-economic circumstances, prolonged unemployment, terrorism, certain aspects of work and the effects of disasters (Taylor 1987) are all topics where more evidence about psychological aspects are necessary in comprehensive studies. Social disadvantage, however defined, leading to inequality of opportunity and poverty should be the concept of such studies, rather than only a specific aspect of it – like unemployment. Interest should be directed not only to the aetiology of the disorder, but to the implications for health services, such as factors producing their poor take-up when provided or inadequate compliance with treatment requirements. Poor use of maternity and child health services by lower socio-economic groups is an important example.

Psychosomatic Disorders

Psychosocial influences on many diseases and disabilities continue to require study. Some such as skin disease, auto-immune disease, or "post-viral" syndromes are likely to be disorders of unknown aetiology and hence, with only symptomatic treatment, of high incidence and of fluctuating course. Even investigation of a physical symptom like incontinence can have an important psychological aspect such as underlying dementia or mood disturbance, or a behavioural factor. More basic studies of the immuno-neuro-endocrine systems in humans are required. Studies should not be confined to this group, but should include virtually any serious disease. Most relevant research has been about the suppression of the immune system, but immune enhancement could now be relevant as in modifying the response to grafts and transplants.

Bio-Psycho-Social Clinical Management

It would be worth reviewing current clinical management of common disorders, where psychological aspects are often implicated in exacerbating distress. Algorithms could be prepared regarding appropriate investigation and treatment, with progress depending on response. Both psychological and pathophysiological aspects require attention, since it would be helpful for any clinician to know how appropriate it would be to pursue standard investigation and treatment in logical steps. The implications for alternative therapies and for decisions about longer term management, such as behaviour therapy, could be considered.

The symptom of pain in its many psychological ramifications also needs further consideration. Pain clinics seem to be mushrooming, often staffed by anaesthetists, yet with the majority of patients presenting with a symptom of unknown aetiology and many of them having psychological disturbances. The role of clinical psychologists in modifying such behaviour has been found to be beneficial; their value, compared with that of other professional staff, should be determined before patterns of such care become too established.

A sensitive psychosocial approach to the caring aspect of stressful diseases like cancer, particularly near to death, has been shown to be of considerable value. Hospice care, whereby there are staff highly experienced in the care of the dying in an environment conducive to taking account of all relevant factors, has wide acceptance, with much appeal for charitable funding. One benefit of this high quality of care is undoubtedly the capability to reduce anxiety and other mood disturbance in both the patient and his family. Even when a physical disorder is static, the patient's distress can fluctuate due to an alteration in psychological response or social support. Hence, in serious chronic disease, assessment needs to be repeated frequently, for clinical management to be dynamic.

Patient Education and Support

There needs to be more exploration of the benefit of relaxation and behaviour modification in the treatment of disease, not least by alternative therapies. Evaluation of various methods which teach the patient self-help would be valuable: manuals could be prepared to assist coping strategies by both the patient and his family. Comparative trials on different methods of providing a modicum of support or sophisticated help are necessary, not least to establish their cost-effectiveness. These should be targeted at clinical management over prolonged periods, such as for coping with severe disability or for establishing simple strategies for problem drinking or cancer counselling. What is the value of relaxation therapy, as provided in its various guises? Why is there increasing demand by patients for such therapies as acupuncture or homeopathy?

How best can information be delivered to individual patients about their treatment and the prevention of complications? What specific factors influence their understanding? The roles and needs of carers require more attention, not least in order to improve their effectiveness and well-being. As long-term management of both psychiatric and physical disorders is transferred more from hospital to community, there is a necessity for a greater understanding about these needs. Even with existing resources, psychological well-being could be improved by better supportive care. Better understanding of the barriers to collaboration, as well as co-operation both between agencies and between individual professional staff are required.

Conclusion

Whatever studies are to be done on the psychological contribution to the causes and course of physical disorders, they must be of impeccable methodology. Far too often, such studies are severely criticised for failing to take account of simple, well-established principles about reliability, validity, sensitivity and specificity in measurement. Much effort can achieve little benefit because of failure e.g. by psychotherapists to follow long-established research requirements, though it must be acknowledged that profound difficulties are involved. These difficulties require more attention, since some excellent studies have been done, for instance on the value of behaviour therapy.

Disablement and disadvantage require as much study of psychological contribution to their cause and course as does disease. It is beyond doubt that psychiatric morbidity is increased with disablement and disadvantage, even though its direct association with disease remains speculative. The severity of psychological and of psychosocial disturbance needs to be established independently and more universally in clinical practice, so that their separate effects can be taken into account.

Mood disturbance, whether anxiety or depression, is to be expected following loss, such as that implied by a diagnosis of cancer. It is important to know the course of adaptation and the pattern of response, in order to respond better, so as to provide relief. Facts are available about pathological responses to grief, but less about, e.g. responses to spinal cord injury. The facts that are known about traumatic amputations, for instance, were mainly based on information concerning war-wounded veterans, and so are very different to those in the common condition today of peripheral vascular disease.

These ideas are intended to be provocative, though some are probably thought to be well studied and understood, and thus not requiring further research. If so, why is the response to need still so inadequate? Too many patients with physical illness suffer as much, if not more, from the emotional reaction to it and its effect on their social circumstances than from the strictly physical effects. Much remains to be done to allow a general understanding that will relieve that aspect of human suffering.

Acknowledgements. I am grateful to my colleagues in Edinburgh, J. W. Affleck, M. Ford, R. J. McGuire, G. Masterton, D. F. Peck, I. Robertson, R. Lewin and M. Brough, who contributed to the discussion from which these ideas emerged.

References

Affleck JW, Aitken RCB, Hunter JAA, McGuire RJ, Roy CW (1988) Rehabilitation status: a measure of medicosocial dysfunction. Lancet I:230–233
Aitken RCB (1969) Measurement of feelings using visual analogue scales. Proc R Soc Med 62:989–993
Aitken RCB (1984) Psychosocial aspects of disease and their management. Psychother Psychosomat 42:55–55
Baker GHB (1987) Psychological factors and immunity. J Psychosom Res 31:1–10
Creed F (1985) Life events and physical illness. J Psychosom Res 29:113–123
Greer S, Morris T, Pettingale K (1979) Psychological response to breast cancer: effect on outcome. Lancet 4:785–787
Johnston DW (1985) Psychological interventions in cardiovascular disease. J Psychosom Res 29:447–456
Lloyd GG (1986) Psychiatric syndromes with a somatic presentation. J Psychosom Res 30:113–120
Mayou R (1986) The psychiatric and social consequence of coronary artery surgery. J Psychosom Res 30:255–271
Meier MJ, Benton AL, Diller L (eds) (1987) Neuro-psychological rehabilitation. Churchill Livingston, Edinburgh
Ron MA (1986) Multiple sclerosis: psychiatric and psychometric abnormalities. J Psychosom Res 30:3–12
Taylor AJ (1987) A taxonomy of disasters and their victims. J Psychosom Res 31:535–544
World Health Organisation (1980) International classification of impairments, disabilities and handicaps. WHO, Geneva

Discussion of Aitken's Report on Psychological Contributions to the Causes and Course of Physical Illness

S. M. Consoli

Introduction

My first observation concerns the ambiguity of the title, which is the "Psychological Contributions to the Causes *and* Course of Physical Illness." In fact, the modes of contribution and mechanisms involved at these two levels of psychosomatic relationships are not comparable, even though they partially overlap. Understanding the first level – that of the psychological causes participating in the triggering of physical illness – supposes that one questions what most specifically determines an individual's somatic vulnerability, when confronted with the stresses of his existence or with emotional constraints. It is not so much a matter of what predisposes an individual to present hypertension instead of a peptic ulcer – as a tendency deriving from Alexander (1950) and the School of Chicago has vainly attempted to prove – but rather, what makes an individual who is faced with a trying life-event fall physically ill, instead of reacting with mental disorders such as anxiety, depression, or psychosis? This question constitutes the basis of psychosomatic research, in the strict sense of the term.

The second level, that of the psychological causes which are instrumental in the course of physical illness, is a much more global aspect. Indeed, the same factors incriminated in the triggering of physical illness may play an important role in its prognosis, but this is also largely dependent on very diverse psychosocial factors, such as the nature of the coping mechanisms used by each subject, the presence of mood disturbances directly or indirectly related to the physical illness, and sometimes the existence of cognitive disorders due to CNS involvement. Other relevant factors are each patient's educational level, his economic resources, the cultural value of the illness within his particular social context, the quality of the social background, etc. This global approach can also be qualified as "psychosomatic", but the use of that term is here much broader and less specific.

Second, the way in which one pursues psychosomatic analysis depends closely on one's aim: does one intend first and foremost to formulate a scientific approach, designed to show the presence of particular cause-and-effect

Centre de Diagnostic, Unité Médico-Psychologique, Hôpital Broussais, 96 Rue Didot, F-75674 Paris Cedex 14

Interaction Between Mental and Physical Illness
Edited by R. Öhman et al.

links and to understand the nature of these links, or, rather, a pragmatic clinical approach, aimed at the optimal planning of care which is best adapted to real needs? Obviously, the two standpoints are not independent, but their imperatives are nonetheless contradictory. The first approach is generally based on a small number of variables, which one attempts to interrelate; the field of study may be a homogeneous category of patients, who are not necessarily representative of the total population presenting the given pathology. For these reasons, extrapolation of results or reproducibility of the research to groups of patients recruited under different conditions may be risky. The utmost care should be paid to ensuring that claimed results are not due to biased sampling – even that which results from the tendency to consult, when within a hospital environment, since such a tendency is well known to be associated with certain specific psychological factors.

Despite these reservations, such selective studies retain the full weight of scientific interest and may well give rise to substantial progress in knowledge of various physical illnesses. The same applies to laboratory studies of healthy subjects, which investigate physiological consequences of the emotions, as a function of each subject's psychological or behavioral characteristics.

On the other hand, the second, more pragmatic approach is related to the notion of therapeutic strategy and economy of health. The questions underlying this approach are as follows:

- How can one best preserve the well-being of a subject presenting physical illness?
- How can one encourage behavioral features likely to improve therapeutic compliance, and combat the features which counter such compliance?
- How can one prevent an illness from becoming a social disadvantage, by mobilizing the most constructive dimensions of the patient's personality?
- How can nonpsychiatric practitioners or even social workers be provided with simple, rapid means of investigation to allow them to measure the degree of "psychological risk" presented by each patient with a physical illness?
- When should one choose a given type of complementary, psychologically orientated treatment, aimed at maximal efficacy but minimal psychological effort and lowest possible financial expense for the patient? The possibilities include psychotropic medication, relaxation, behavioral therapy, supportive psychotherapy, and psychoanalytical psychotherapy.

Evaluation of Coping Mechanisms

Although numerous authors agree on the value of studies of coping mechanisms in patients who present with physical illness, much remains to be done for such an evaluation to be reliable, valid, and sensitive. Work by Lazarus (1966) has led to the establishment of a useful scale, but current diffusion of it remains limited. Ray et al. (1982) have developed an interesting classification of coping mechanisms, based on the following two dimensions: on the one hand, the subject's acknowledgement or disavowal of the perception of threat, experienced harm or challenge, related to the stressful situation; on the other hand, the subject's degree of control or helplessness, when faced with the same stressful situation. It is thus possible to describe successively a series of coping mechanisms, designated by the terms: rejection, concern for control, and resignation as regards acknowledgement of the threat, and minimization, avoidance, and dependency, as regards rejection of the threat.

Nevertheless, several questions have yet to be answered: How can the intensity of each of these coping mechanisms be measured most reliably? Is the patient's answer to a questionnaire sufficient? Is not the test itself a stressful situation, to which the subject will react by defending himself, according to his capacities, and by giving a deformed image of his true behavior?

Moreover, is there a relationship between the coping mechanisms the subject brings into play, when confronted with the stress of illness, and his general behavior when faced with the stresses of his existence, or even with his behavior before falling physically ill?

Finally, there are obviously no "good" and "bad" coping mechanisms, even though certain attitudes appear more rigid than others, or certain attitudes suppose a more intensive adaptation effort on the part of the subject. Indeed, the most important factor is the result provided by the coping mechanisms: are they effective or ineffective? Do they succeed in controlling anxiety or not? Do they leave the subject with a sensation of having a certain freedom to maneuver, even if he chooses to resign himself to fate or to other persons, or does the subject live his reactions as though he had no choice?

A fascinating subsidiary question is that of the possible relationship between certain categories of coping mechanisms and certain types of physiological reactions: the adrenal medulla, the hypothalamic adrenal cortex axis, the secretion of epinephrine and norepinephrine, secretion by the various endocrine glands, and immunomodulation chiefly involving the T or B lymphocytes are solicited in various ways, according to whether the subject is confronted with escapable or inescapable stress, and according to whether he adopts an overall attitude of defence or of defeat. It would be most interesting to study this observation in depth, by conducting methodologically rigorous experimental works. Perhaps it would thus be possible to confirm certain hypotheses put forward several years ago, by such authors as Alexander or Dunbar seeking an analogy between the induced psychic conflicts and the physiological functions involved in various physical illnesses.

Capacity to Take Advantage of Social Support

We are obliged to recognize that there is no parallelism between the importance of social support existing in the friends and family of a subject who is ill, and the use to which the latter puts this support. Naturally, the lack of such support constitutes a pejorative prognostic index, in the course of any pathology. One of the most exemplary studies on this subject is that by Ruberman et al. (1984) on mortality subsequent to myocardial infarction. But it is obvious that certain subjects may behave as though they were alone, despite their being well surrounded in reality. These subjects continue to live shut up in their conflicts, unable to express their distress to others, or ask for genuine help; moreover, in some cases, the greater the insistence with which help is proposed, the more adamant their refusal of it.

Birtchnell (1981) has proposed a judicious classification of interpersonal relationships, based on a bi-dimensional description, which takes into account the attachment to or detachment from others, and the tendency towards directiveness or receptiveness in an exchange situation. Thus, dependent behavior may be considered to be the result of a need for attachment and closeness, combined with a need for receptivity and passivity. In this manner, one can describe altruistic or even possessive personalities, who look after others but dislike being looked after themselves, or dominant and aloof personalities, who like directing but prefer to maintain a distance. Such classifications seem to be very useful, in conjunction with the study of coping mechanisms, for evaluating the adaptation capacity of a subject faced with the trial of undergoing a physical illness. They may even be useful for determining the degree of vulnerability of subjects who remain in good health as long as they are not confronted with excessive stresses, or as long as they have the impression of maintaining a certain freedom in the handling of their interpersonal relationships.

Comparative Studies Between Various Clinical Categories

Serious methodological problems arise when one attempts to apply the psychological measurements, carried out on a study population, to the physical disease characterizing the given population, even when such variables as age, sex, sociocultural level, conditions of the examination, etc. are taken into account. The choice of a control population always presents major difficulties: it does not allow a distinction to be drawn between the psychological etiological factors of the physical disease and the psychological repercussions of the disease. The latter must always be taken into account, even for pathologies which do not call the prognosis for life into play, and which engender neither functional disablement nor a psychosocial handicap. Indeed, the mere fact of being labelled ill, e.g., in cases of hypertension, gives rise to moral discomfort, which varies from one subject to the next. The comparison of diseases is no easier a task, since each differs in terms of its symptomatological expression and cultural image, from which its psychological repercussions derive. There is thus enormous value in comparing subjects belonging to clinically similar subgroups in terms of the consulting symptom, but in which etiology is of varying severity. This is the case for a highly demonstrative study by Wirsching et al. (1982) in females with mammary tumors, investigated prior to biopsy. This is also the case for a study we conducted recently in a group of patients presenting Raynaud's phenomenon, and examined for etiological determination upon admission to hospital. At the time of the trial, the patients did not yet know the outcome of their examination, in favor of idiopathic Raynaud's disease, a benign disorder, or Raynaud's secondary phenomenon, which is most often of sclerodermal origin and thus constitutes a more serious prognosis. Such examples represent elegant demonstrations of the possible links between fragility of psychic functioning and severity or organic involvement in the course of illness.

Longitudinal Studies on Patients Belonging to Risk Groups

One of the most convincing ways of testing hypotheses derived from experimental works or from observation of a clinical group is to follow up the clinical course of patients belonging to a risk group. Such patients should be monitored over a sufficiently long period for the cumulative incidence of a specific disease to attain a valid percentage of the initial population. Depending on the cases, this supposes either that the morbid risk be very clear, or that the study be of long duration, resulting in loss to follow up of a nonnegligible number of subjects, and presenting major difficulties for interpretation of the epidemiological measurements.

The risk factors studied have not been limited to alcoholism or tobacco dependence. The clinical course of ischemic cardiopathy patients subsequent to a first myocardial infarction has been examined many times, for example. However, there have been few studies of borderline hypertensives, and more systematic research is required in the area of precancerous lesions. A psychosomatic approach is fully justified in the domain of seropositivity to the HIV virus: are subjects who develop AIDS psychologically comparable to others? Is the rapidity of onset of signs of ARC or AIDS related to psychological or behavioral factors?

Such studies are complex in methodological terms, since the most psychologically vulnerable subjects of a biologically exposed group generally present behavioral disorders which may be instrumental in the course of the physical disease or the onset of a complication. This is the case with noncompliance with dietetic rules in vascular risk subjects and with the multiplication of further contamination or even delayed treatment or opportunist infections in HIV seropositives.

How Should the Observer's Position Be Taken into Account?

The concern with reproducibility of a psychological or behavioral observation and the desire to use reliable measuring instruments often leads investigators to consider the observer's position as a confounding variable needing to be eliminated or at least experimentally controlled. This honorable scientific objective is a necessary condition if the observer has an a priori idea of possible findings, and if knowledge of certain clinical characteristics, such as the presence or absence of a physical disorder, risks biasing the evaluation of psychological features.

Even when the studied data are based on the subjects' replies rather than on the investigator's evaluation, it is known that the way in which a questionnaire is presented or a psychological test is justified, or the way in which subjects' participation is motivated may substantially affect the results obtained. This factor is often neglected, and may account as much for the false links between variables as for the absence of a significant link, given massive variability in the "observer" factor. It has likewise been maintained that the severity of the alexithymic phenomena observed during psychosomatic investigation may be related to the anxiety caused by examination conditions, and to the subject's resorting to a coping mechanism to protect him from the observer's intrusion. Whatever the case, it may well be interesting in a psychosomatic approach to consider the observer's position not as a confounding, but as a capital variable. Indeed, the psychological effect produced on the observer, his "counter-transferential" emotional reactions, and the impression of closeness or distance produced by the subject, all constitute particularly useful indices of the subject's mental functioning and of his capacity to enter into relationships with others. The more the observer's evaluation is taken into account, the less reproducible, but at the same time the more complete the study, in that it more reliably accounts for the observed subject's psychosomatic equilibrium.

Can One Reconcile the Observation of Behavior and the Taking into Account of Unconscious Functioning, in Keeping with a Psychoanalytical Model?

This is a complex problem, since it is very dangerous to seek to draw general rules from clinical material collected in the course of psychotherapeutic or psychoanalytical treatment of patients with organic disorders, or of neurotic patients presenting a somatic episode during therapy. Certain of these observations are nevertheless very subtle, and should be carefully examined. At the other extreme, behavioral approaches may appear scientifically much more rigorous, but often yield conclusions which are too general or too approximate, and whose scope may appear very limited in comparison with the investment in setting up the studies.

Numerous French authors remain faithful to the psychoanalytical model and ascribe major importance to unconscious conflicts and ego-defence mechanisms in the emotional disturbances at the root of much organic pathology. Thus, the notion of alexithymia formulated by Nemiah et al. (1976; see also Apfel and Sifneos 1979), with its possible neurophysiological implications, has its counterpart in the notion of *pensée opératoire* formulated by Marty (1980), related to the inhibition of representational activity and to a limitation of fantasy life. According to various authors with psychoanalytical training, the suppression of affect, notably anxiety and aggressive drives, plays a fundamental role in the somatic vulnerability of numerous patients: such suppression can be considered as both the effect and the result of inhibition of fantasy life. Certain measuring instruments, such as Hackett and Cassem's Denial Scale (1974), the Hostility and Direction of Hostility Questionnaire, or Beth Israel Hospital's alexithymic scale, allow partial apprehension of the suppression of affect. However, these do not replace projective personality tests such as the Rorschach or Murray's Thematic Apperception Test (TAT), the former now including standardized rating criteria, due in particular, to work by Exner (1986). Both these tests constitute sensitive means for observing an individual's latent tendencies, his capacity to elaborate conflicts, and his means for representing anxiety and freeing himself from the impact of trauma through the possibilities offered by symbolization.

Consequently, works exploiting the combined results of several categories of instruments are most desirable; these instruments may bring into play behavioral, psychoanalytical, or physiological and biological approaches. The result should be improved determination of the common elements, and thereby, the formulation of more pertinent criteria for psychosomatic study.

References

Alexander F (1950) Psychosomatic medicine. Norton, New York

Apfel RJ, Sifneos PE (1979) Alexithymia: concept and measurement. Psychother Psychosom 32:180–190

Birtchnell J (1987) Attachment-detachment, directiveness-receptiveness: a system for classifying interpersonal attitudes and behaviour. Br J Med Psychol 60:17–27

Consoli S, Bayle O, Baudin M, Fiessinger JN, Vayssairat M, Housset E (1986) Clinical evaluation of personality of patients presenting Raynaud's phenomenon. Psychiatrie et Psychobiologie 1:288–297

Consoli S, Bayle O, Baudin M, Fiessinger JN, Vayssairat M, Housset E (1987) Distinctive attitudes to the Rosenzweig test in subjects presenting idiopathic or secondary Raynaud's phenomenon. Psychiatrie et Psychobiologie 2:42–50

Exner JE (1986) The Rorschach: a comprehensive system, vol 1: basic foundations. Wiley, New York

Hackett TP, Cassem NH (1974) Development of a quantitative rating scale to assess denial. J Psychosom Res 18:93–100

Lazarus RS (1966) Psychological stress and the coping process. McGraw-Hill, New York

Marty P (1980) L'ordre psychosomatique. Désorganisation et régressions. Payot, Paris

Nemiah JC, Freyberger H. Sifneos PE (1976) Alexithymia: a view of the psychosomatic process. In: Hill O (ed) Modern trends in psychosomatic medicine, vol 3. Butterworths, London

Ray C, Lindop J, Gibson S (1982) The concept of coping. Psychol Med 12:385–395

Ruberman W, Weinblatt E, Goldberg JD, Chaudhary BS (1984) Psychosocial influences on mortality after myocardial infarction. N Engl J Med 311:552–559

Wirsching M, Stierlin H, Hoffman F, Weber G, Wirsching B (1982) Psychological identification of breast cancer patients before biopsy. J Psychosom Res 26:1–10

Behavioral Aspects of Physical Illness

K. G. GÖTESTAM

The area of behavioral aspects of physical illness is a vast one: it includes the old definition of psychosomatic disorders, but is broader, in the sense of comprehending all psychological factors contributing to the etiology, maintenance, treatment, and prevention of illness. According to Engel (1986) behavior is defined as "All responses (physical, cognitive, overt behavior) on illness, leading to or prior to illness."

Behavioral medicine, then, is the application of current behavioral knowledge to the entire medical field. In practice, the denotations psychological medicine, health psychology, and behavioral medicine are more or less synonymous. It is impossible to cover the entire field here, but the general framework and some illustrative cases will pe presented.

State of the Art

Behavior and Physical Illness

Can behavior really affect physical health or lead to physical illness? In several areas, it is now evident that behavior or lifestyle may include health hazards and may affect illness: passivity can lead to obesity, overeating to diabetes, alcohol consumption to hypertension, smoking to cancer, and type-A behavior patterns to coronary heart disease.

Behavior Change and Physical Illness

When behavior changes, changes can also result in physical illness (e.g. hypertension, obesity), and even change the incidence of physical illness (Puska 1973; Puska et al. 1978).

In the behavioral treatment of physical illness, instruction is a significant aspect, but the instructions have to be very concrete and elaborated in detail, forming a management plan; the simple instruction "Keep your blood pressure

---

Produced at Stanford University. Present address:
Department of Psychiatry and Behavioural Medicine, University of Trondheim, Östmarka Hospital, P.O. Box 3008 Lade, N-7002 Trondheim

Interaction Between Mental and Physical Illness
Edited by R. Öhman et al.

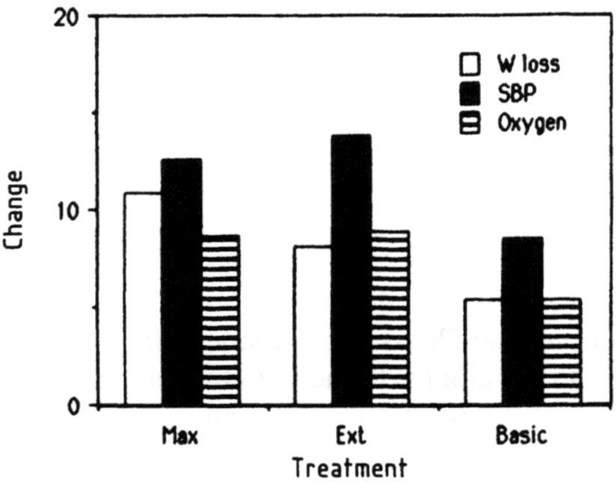

Fig. 1. Reduction of coronary heart disease risk for 75 high-risk patients through an 8-week behavioral treatment program (at three levels – maximum, extended, and basic). The data reported are on weight loss, systolic blood pressure, and aerobic capacity (data from Lovibond et al. 1986)

low" has in fact been shown to be counter-productive (Suls et al. 1986). Thus, the doctor's activity level is of relatively little value, while the practical advice to the patient is of the utmost importance. This finding has been shown consistently in several studies of psychosomatic disorders. The doctor's knowledge of the illness and contact with the patient are not enough, although they may have some effect on the illness: the important issue is the way the problems encountered by the patient are managed.

In a study by Lovibond et al. (1986), an 8-week behavioral program (at three levels – maximal, extended, and basic) was implemented for 75 patients who were at high risk for coronary heart disease (CHD). The program included training in several aspects which were thought to be important for this CHD risk. All three levels were effective in reducing the risk of CHD with regard to weight change, blood pressure, and aerobic capacity (Fig. 1).

Behavioral Approaches to Somatic Illness

Several behavioral approaches have been used to improve somatic treatment techniques, both pharmacotherapeutical and surgical methods.

Patient Compliance or Adherence

When a patient has malignant hypertension, he is in great need of medication, but some patients "forget" the pills and are only partially compliant with the treatment regimen, producing a severe health hazard for themselves. Different procedures have been used to improve adherence, including the use of signals or cues, practicing application of the medication (particularly for diabetic patients), structuring the environment to facilitate the medication regimen, and giving various forms of rewards for adhering to the regimen.

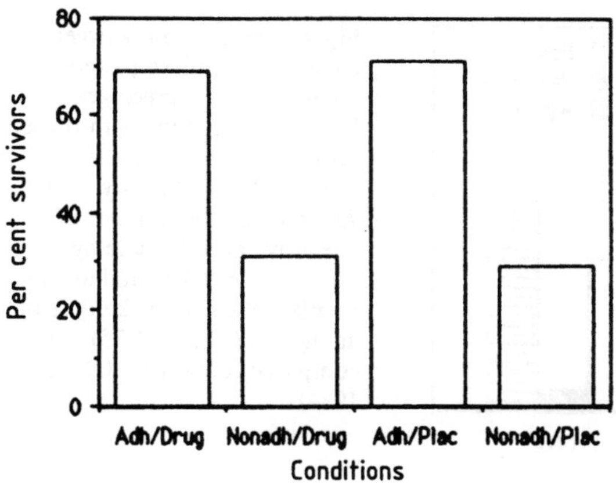

Fig. 2. The effect of adherence to a drug regimen in the Coronary Drug Project, where clofibrate was shown to result in fewer survivors than placebo, and adherers survived more than nonadherers (data from the Coronary Drug Project 1980)

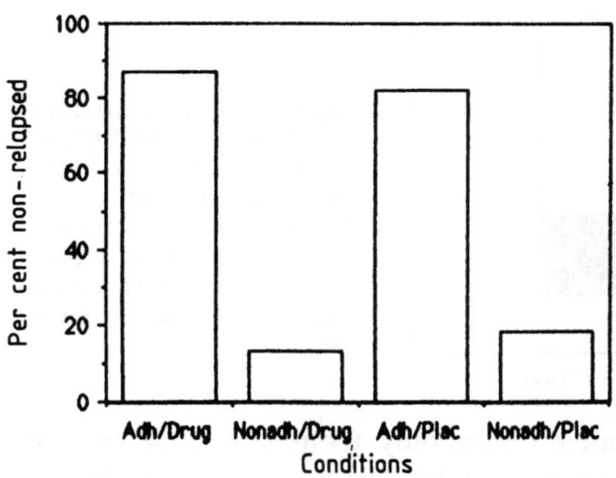

Fig. 3. The effect of adherence to a drug regimen in a Schizophrenia Drug Project, where neuroleptic drugs were shown to result in fewer relapses than placebo, and adherers had fewer relapses than nonadherers (data from Hogarty et al. 1973)

In the Coronary Drug Project (1980) clofibrate was found to be very toxic, leaving more survivors on the placebo treatment than on the drug. An important result, however, was, that adherence to the regimen was found to be more important for the outcome than the drug itself (see Fig. 2).

Similarly, in a schizophrenia drug project (Hogarty et al. 1973), adherence to taking the drug was more important than the effect of the drug (Fig. 3).

However, both these studies had several weaknesses. Probably the most important was the question of what selection could be working on the different groups, since adherence was not implemented by the researchers, but only studied. Thus, the studies were not experimental in design. There are, however, several recent publications reporting specific study of adherence, with by and large the same results (see Melamed and Siegel 1980, for a review).

Maintenance

For the cessation of smoking several different treatment strategies have been reported to make almost 100% of subjects smoke-free immediately after com-

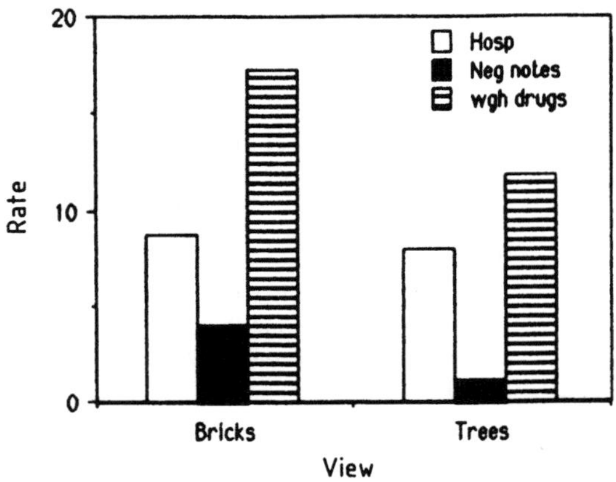

Fig. 4. Comparison between cholecystectomized patients seeing trees and green grass from their window, with those only seeing a brick wall. Length of hospital stay (8.70, 7.96 days), total number of "negative notes" made by nurses (3.96, 1.13), and average number of daily weak doses of analgesics (17.31, 11.75) are compared (data from Ulrich 1984)

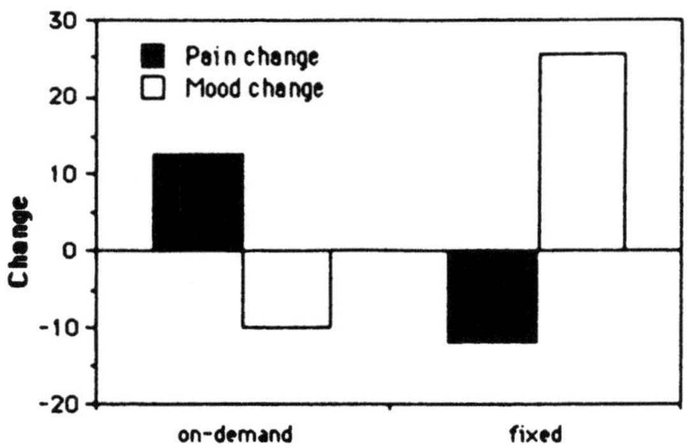

Fig. 5. Comparison between a time-contingent (fixed-time) and a pain-contingent (PRN, on-demand) medication schedule of analgesic drugs given to a population of patients with chronic pain (data from Berntzen and Götestam 1987)

pletion of the treatment, but after 1 year, only about 15%–30% were still smoke-free (Schwartz 1987). The effective long-term treatment of smoking, therefore, seems to remain an issue unresolved so far. In the treatment of alcoholism, however, good results have been reported in the maintenance of gains by the Relapse Prevention Model (Marlatt and Gordon 1985). This model includes social skills training to allow maintenance of the patient's status as abstinent or as a controlled drinker.

Management

The setting in which the patient is treated may be of importance for outcome. In a study by Ulrich (1984), the recovery of cholecystectomized patients was better in those who were in a room with a pleasant view of trees and green grass, compared with those who only saw a brick wall (see Fig. 4).

The timing of medication also has its effects, apart from the purely pharmacological ones. Berntzen and Götestam (1987) varied the schedule for a group of patients with chronic pain: they received their usual analgesic drug, but in one period on-demand (PRN, pain-contingent) and in another period with a fixed time-table. The results showed clear improvements both in pain and mood with fixed time, but were worse with the on-demand schedule (Fig. 5).

Health Promotion

Several programs have used a number of approaches to improve the general state of health of populations (Puska 1973; Puska et al. 1983). These are further discussed below.

Behavioral Treatment Procedures for Somatic Illness

Behavioral treatment procedures have been developed for many somatic illnesses, viz. (a) chronic pain, (b) epilepsy, (c) hypertension, (d) coronary heart disease, (e) immunity and cancer, (f) diabetes, (g) asthma, (h) insomnia, (i) headache, (j) Raynaud's disease, (k) arthritis, (l) gastritis or peptic ulcer, (m) skin diseases, and (n) stroke rehabilitation (for a review, see Yates 1980). A few examples will be presented here.

Chronic Pain

Linton and Götestam (1985) have shown in an operant analogue study that a pain response can be developed and maintained, even when the noxious stimulus has disappeared: this became a model for the development of chronic pain (see Fig. 6). They also have shown (1984) in a clinical population with

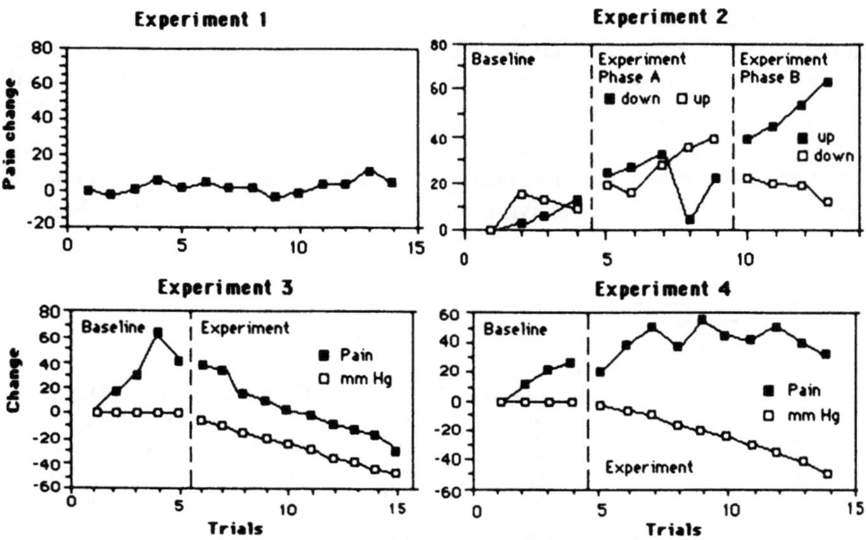

Fig. 6. An operant analogue to test the development and maintenance of pain responses even when the noxious stimulus has disappeared. In Experiment 1, constant stimulation and no feedback were given; in Experiment 2, constant stimulation, and positive feedback (on either increase or decrease in pain responses); in Experiment 3, decreased pain stimulation and no feedback; and in Experiment 4, decreased pain stimulation and positive feedback on increased pain reports – "the chronic pain analogue" (data from Linton and Götestam 1985)

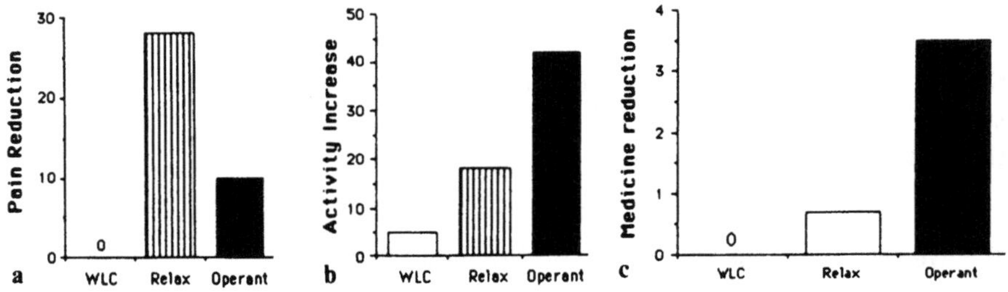

Fig. 7. Treatment of chronic pain patients with either a relaxation procedure or an operant approach. The relaxation procedure was most effective on subjective pain (**a**), while the operant procedure was effective in increasing activity (**b**) and reducing medication (**c**) (data from Linton and Götestam 1984)

chronic pain that an operant procedure is effective in increasing activity and reducing medication, whereas a relaxation procedure is more effective in reducing the subjective experience of pain (Fig. 7).

Epilepsy

Dahl et al. (1985) treated 18 children with an extensive behavioral analysis, followed by teaching the child, parents, and teachers to observe preseizure events and then to reinforce seizure control techniques and healthy behavior. The results showed a clear improvement in the treatment group, while the control group became worse in the long run (Fig. 8). Another study (Dahl et al. 1987) of 18 adult epileptic patients presented similar results: improvement occurred in the treatment group and the waiting-list control group showed no change, whereas the control group receiving only attention became worse (see Fig. 9).

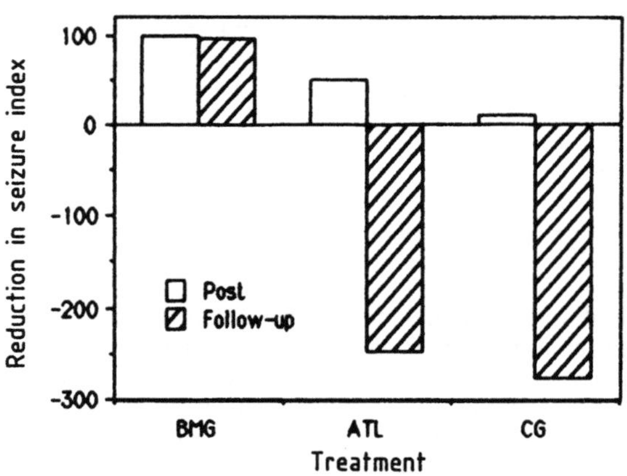

Fig. 8. Results from the treatment of 18 children with refractory epilepsy. The figure illustrates the reduction from pretreatment to posttreatment and 1 year follow-up, for the behavior therapy group, an attention control group, and a control group (data from Dahl et al. 1985)

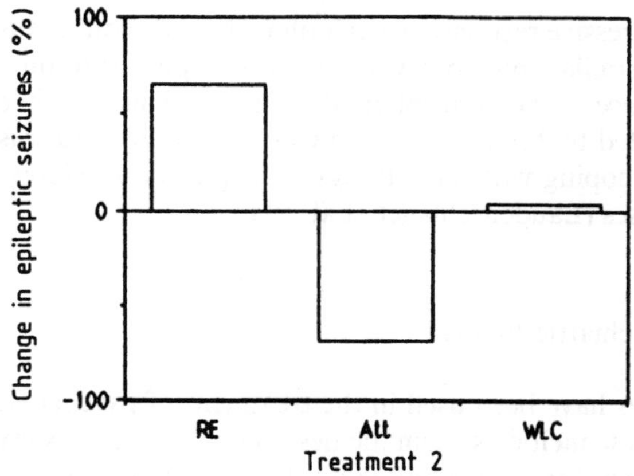

Fig. 9. Results from the treatment of 18 adults with refractory epilepsy. The figure illustrates the reduction from pretreatment to 10 weeks' post-treatment, for the behavior therapy group, an attention control group, and a waiting-list control group (data from Dahl et al. 1987)

Hypertension

Normal persons are generally flexible in their blood pressure, while hypertensive patients are less flexible: it is unclear what effect psychological intervention may have in this connection. Roccella et al. (1986) have stated that only three factors are clearly of importance: weight control, alcohol restriction (<2 oz./day), and sodium restriction (<2 g/day). On the other hand, caffeine/nicotine, nutrition, exercise, relaxation/biofeedback, do not show such clear effects. They also stated that "all patients should be included in some kind of behavioural treatment."

Immunity and Cancer

In a series of animal studies by Ader and Cohen (1975), it was shown that the immune function could be easily conditioned by the conditioned taste aversion

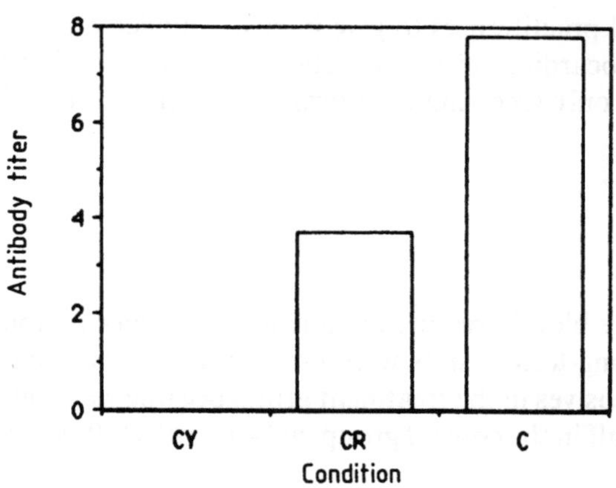

Fig. 10. An experiment for the evaluation of conditioning of immune suppression by cyclophosphamide (CY) in a one-trial learning conditioned taste aversion paradigm. The response on CY is shown at the *left* of the figure, the conditioned response after only the taste stimulus in the *middle*, and on the *left* the response after only the taste stimulus in rats not trained in a conditioning trial (data from Ader and Cohen 1977)

procedure. The immunosuppressive response to cyclophosphamide could thus be conditioned, resulting in similar, but somewhat weaker responses to only the taste stimulus in the absence of cyclophosphamide (Fig. 10). This principle had already been demonstrated by Metal'nikov and Chorine (1926), and was later shown to be related to coping with such things as helplessness, widowhood, and other kinds of losses (Laudenschlager et al. 1983).

Behavioral Treatment in Psychiatric Illness

Several behavioral techniques have been used in the treatment of psychiatric illness (Leitenberg 1976). These include systematic desensitization for anxiety and phobia, exposure treatment for phobia and panic disorder, exposure with response prevention for obsessive-compulsive disorder, cognitive therapy for depression, token economy for schizophrenia, and operant procedures for sexual disorders, anorexia nervosa, bulimia, and dementia. In addition, there are several methods for the treatment of addictive disorders, such as social-skills training procedures for alcoholism, drug addiction, and smoking (Melin and Götestam 1980).

Behavioral Community Approaches

Special large-scale community intervention programs have been implemented to reduce smoking, hypertension, and cardiovascular risks. In many of the cardiovascular programs, treatment of both smoking and hypertension have also been included, as they are among the main risk factors.

Smoking

Burt et al. (1974) asked general practitioners to give intensive advice on how to give up smoking to postmyocardial infarction patients who were visiting them. Compared with patients only receiving the normal care, this improved the results from 28% to 62%.

Hypertension

In a large-scale project to reduce blood pressure in patients with hypertension at the Lockheed factory, the long-term results were promising, showing that about 60% of high-risk hypertensives in the treatment group became well controlled, compared with about half in the control group, at 24 months follow-up (Agras et al. 1986).

Cardiovascular Risk

In the National Pepsico Trial, the aim was to reduce cardiovascular risk at the work site. Of four sites, with 400 workers each, two underwent intervention, and two served as controls: the preliminary results (C. Barr Taylor, personal communication) show significant reductions in cholesterol, blood pressure, and cigarette smoking in the experimental but not in the control groups.

At the Stanford Heart Disease Prevention Program, similar results have been gained in respect of smoking, overweight, hypertension, heart disease and total morbidity, but not cholesterol levels (C. Barr Taylor, personal communication).

Use of Computers in Treatment and Research

Computers have recently become very useful in medicine both for clinical work and research.

Diagnosis

Different programs can be used on a personal computer (PC) to score rating scales and questionnaires directly without having to use paper and pencil, and then code the results.

Expert Systems

Through expert systems, it is now possible to load a PC with information, and have it answer different questions, as a decision-tree for diagnosis or treatment (e.g. DSM-III).

Computer-Assisted Therapy

In a study by Burnett et al. (1985), patients were given a pocket calculator to record the amount eaten, and amount exercised, and they received specific feedback on this information. This procedure was shown to be effective during the 8-week treatment program, but even more at 6 months follow-up.

In a video-assisted program for obesity, Saylor (1987) used video first to give detailed instructions on how to reduce weight, but most importantly to lead the patients back to the instructions when the program was functioning less well. He reported superior results compared with other behavioral programs for obesity at 3 and 6 months, and even improved results at the 4-month follow-up.

Educational Programmes

Special visual programs can be prepared, and used by patients to give them education in specific areas, for instance, alcoholism. The PC can be loaded with alternative program pieces, so that an individual patient can have specific feedback on his/her specific answers.

Electronic Mail Systems

Through the university data networks (i.e., Bitnet, Earn), it is possible to be in contact with researchers throughout the world, within minutes. It is possible to send either short messages, long data files, or manuscripts.

Electronic Scientific Journals

A scientific journal, SPUR, "Scandinavian Psychiatric Update & Research", reachable through the data mail systems, or simple phone modems, will be introduced in 1988 (with the present author as editor).

Research Planning

A Research Model

A viable research model is necessary to investigate causal relationships effectively. Brownell (1982) has presented such a model (Fig. 11), which has been used to look at coronary heart disease (Fig. 12) and lung cancer (Fig. 13). In it, the causal relationships are investigated stepwise, ending with interventions to reduce the incidence of the illness. Both examples have been used extensively, and with relatively good results – though possibly not satisfactory on the clinical level, since sufficiently effective interventions are still lacking, but clear enough to prove the usefulness and logic of the model.

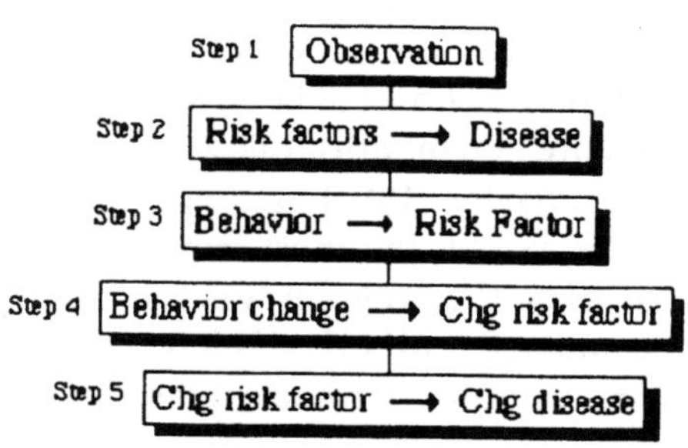

Fig. 11. A research model for the investigation of causal relationships in behavioral medicine (from Brownell 1984)

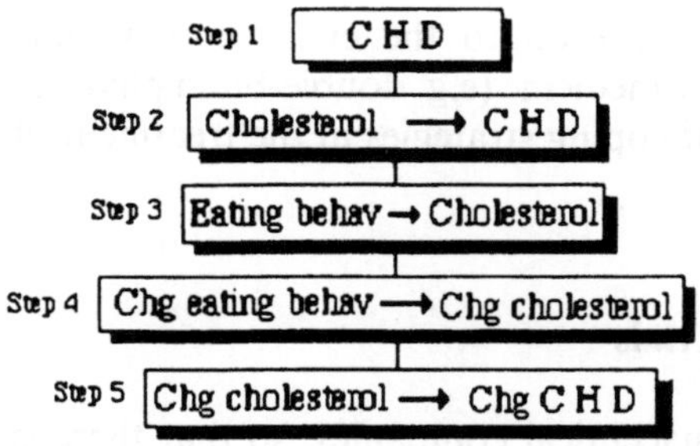

Fig. 12. Application of a research model for the investigation of causal relationships on coronary heart disease

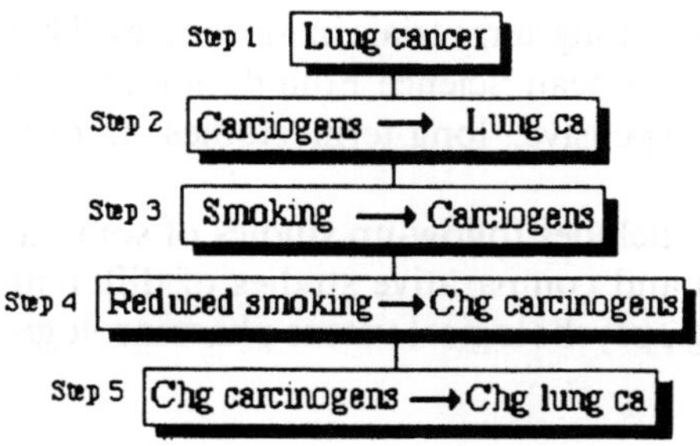

Fig. 13. Application of a research model for the investigation of causal relationships on lung cancer

All steps include careful observation, while in addition, steps 4 and 5 have an intervention character, and can lead to prevention of illness. The model emphasizes the understanding of etiology, while the necessary empirical research on intervention is being performed.

A Bio-Behavioral Approach

Both psychological factors such as learning and biological factors are important and necessary ingredients in an effective approach. Too many psychologists neglect biology, and too many doctors neglect psychology. The psychiatrist should use both.

Intervention Research

Development and evaluation of intervention strategies are important both in the short and long term. In the short-term perspective, we need to know more about the effects of the interventions we are currently using, and we are also in great need of new techniques. In the long run, this kind of research is important for the understanding of theoretical issues.

Behavioral strategies are also useful in research, and several new areas could be of interest to improve the evaluation of current treatment techniques, e.g., in surgery. Totally new diseases, such as acquired immune deficiency syndrome (AIDS), should also be the subject of such research.

Research is needed particularly in relation to the evaluation of psychosocial interventions in psychosomatic medicine (e.g. double-blind pharmacological trials) and the development of coping strategies in the treatment of physical illness.

Long-Term Treatment and Prevention Trials

Many drug trials are funded by pharmaceutical companies, so that there is limited financing and a primary clinical-practical aim. Funding from national research boards is also insufficient to allow long-term trials in most cases. This is probably an important task for the European Science Foundation and its associated organizations: to support expensive, long-term studies in psychosocial interventions.

Research that is needed in this area includes follow-up studies of somatic treatment for psychosomatic disorders and comparative studies of different treatment approaches or modalities (e.g., psychological versus pharmacological).

Reimbursement for Health Care

Sternbach (1974) has called one type of chronic patient the "professional patient": this is one who gets paid to be sick and show symptoms, i.e., with a disability pension.

This problem is closely related to the strategy of prescribing bedrest for pain: is there in fact a relationship between pain and activity? Linton (1985) has looked at this question and found that in a global sense, there is a high correlation, but the closer the activity is observed, the less is the correlation (Fig. 14).

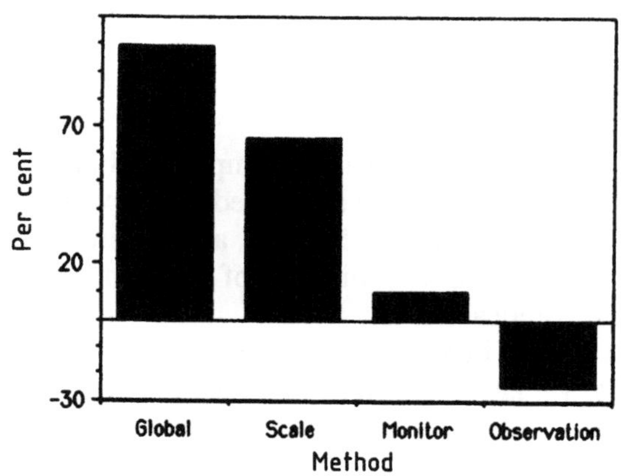

Fig. 14. The correlations between pain and activity in a group of chronic pain patients, related to the degree of concreteness of the assessment. With global evaluation, the correlation is high, with thorough observation, it is negative (data from Linton 1985)

Nachemson (1985) has stated that the patient with chronic pain will be best off if s/he goes back to work as soon as possible. Deyo et al. (1986) have compared patients who were randomly assigned to 2-day or 7-day bedrest, respectively, for lower back pain. The 2-day strategy was better with regard to absenteeism from work, as expected, but it also led to less pain.

Loss of activity usually lead to misery: satisfaction in work is a more important factor than workload, which has no predictive power for the development of chronic pain states (Nachemson 1985). Albert Camus has said that: "without work, all life will soon decay, but if the work is without a soul, it will slowly choke to death."

Research is needed here into the effects of reimbursement/disability payments (patient activity/work, social functioning, quality of life).

Cost-Effectiveness

Liaison psychiatry and its associated research are no longer popular among somatic doctors. Related to this is the fact that people often turn to traditional medicine, chaplains, and nonprofessionals, instead of asking for advice from psychiatry. There have been, however, some recent attempts to change this picture, specifically within the framework of behavioral medicine.

Smith et al. (1986) have studied psychiatric consultation in somatization disorder. They invited general practitioners to participate, and these doctors were randomized: in the experimental group, patient referrals resulted in a letter with specific advice to the doctor. Somatization Disorder was thoroughly described, including its chronic relapsing course and low mortality and morbidity rates. These doctors were also encouraged to act as primary physician for the patients, and recommendations were also included for management. Regular appointments were suggested at intervals of 4–6 weeks to avoid patients having to acquire and show symptoms to be allowed to meet the doctor. It was recommended that the visits should always include a physical check-up, but admission to hospital, elaborate diagnostic procedures, and laboratory assessments, as well as surgical intervention should be avoided. The doctor should not say "It's all in your head."

After some time, a crossover of the doctors was made, and the control group was now given the same instructions as the experimental group had been given before. The results showed a drastic reduction in the number of hospital days for the experimental group, and a similar reduction during the intervention period (period 2) for the control group (Fig. 15). Also, the total health care was drastically reduced.

Maguire et al. (1982) have implemented a study of a counselling service to women undergoing mastectomy: one nurse gave this counselling, both before and after operation, and she also monitored the patients' progress. As shown in Fig. 16, total costs of management went down (the nurse's salary being included in the costs for the experimental group). This was the case both for

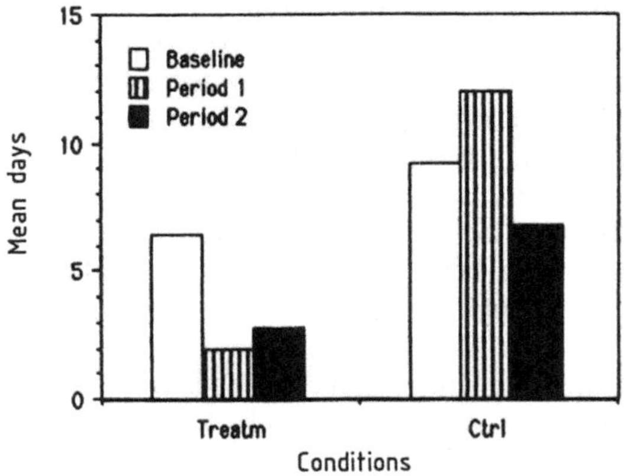

Fig. 15. Mean number of hospital days per year for patients with somatization disorder. The treatment group consists of GPs randomized to the experimental condition, and the control group of doctors who were crossed-over to intervention in period 2. Periods 1 and 2 were each 9 months (data from Smith et al. 1986)

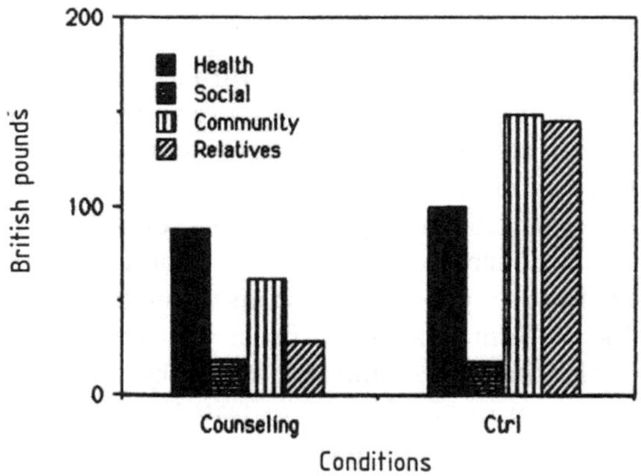

Fig. 16. Total health, social, community, and family costs for women undergoing mastectomy. The costs for the nurse giving the counselling service and the monitoring of the project are included in health costs in the counselling group (data from Maguire et al. 1982)

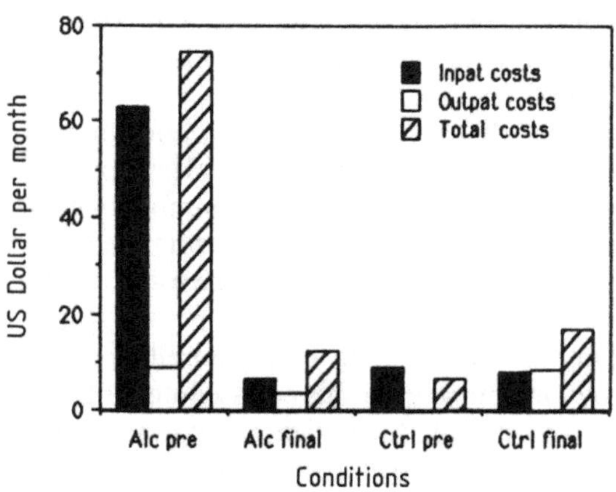

Fig. 17. Costs for health service to alcoholics in the alcohol group and a nonalcohol control group during the 4-year project period (data from Holder and Hallan 1981)

health costs (psychiatric and other hospital costs), community costs, and expenses for the relatives.

In California, Holder and Hallan (1981) have studied the cost and utilization of medical care during a 5-year alcohol treatment project (under the health insurance system), aimed at giving a uniform treatment service to alcoholics, who had previously had very varying resources available to them. The goal was to give acute inpatient care about 6 days per year, intermediate inpatient care 21 days per year, residential care 30 days per year, and outpatient care 45 times per year. The program included a 2-year intervention program plus 2-year follow-up.

There was a rapid increase in utilization of care during the first year, but it then settled down at a lower level. Both effectiveness and utilization were increased, and eventually this also reduced the overall costs (Fig. 17).

Under this heading the research needed includes cost-effectiveness studies on chronic diseases – symptoms, social functioning, hobbies, working capacity, working years gained during a lifetime, and quality of life.

Acknowledgement. Information and help in the preparation of the manuscript from several colleagues is gratefully acknowledged, especially from W. Stewart Agras and C. Barr Taylor at Stanford University. The preparation of this manuscript was supported in part by the Medical Faculty of the University of Trondheim and the Norwegian Research Board for Science and the Humanities (project number 13.35.65-003)

References

Ader R, Cohen N (1977) Behaviorally conditioned immunosuppression. Psychosom Med 37:333–340

Agras WS, Taylor CB, Kraemer HC, Southam MA, Schneider JA (1986) Relaxation training for essential hypertension at the worksite: II. The poorly controlled hypertensive. Psychosom Med 49:264–273

Berntzen D, Götestam KG (1987) Effects of on-demand or fixed interval schedules in the treatment of chronic pain with analgesic compounds: an experimental comparison. J Consult Clin Psychol 55:213–217

Brownell KD (1982) Behavioral medicine. Annu Rev Behav Ther Theory Pract 8:156–207

Burnett KF, Taylor CB, Agras WS (1985) Ambulatory computer-assisted therapy for obesity: a new frontier for behavior therapy. J Consult Clin Psychol 53:698–703

Burt A, Thornley P, Illingworth D, White P, Shaw TRD, Turner R (1974) Stopping smoking after myocardial infarction. Lancet I:304–306

Coronary Drug Project Research Group (1980) Influence of adherence to treatment and response of cholesterol on mortality in the Coronary Drug Project. N Engl J Med 303:1038–1041

Dahl JA, Melin L, Brorson LO, Schollin J (1985) Effects of a broad-spectrum behavior modification treatment program on children with refractory epileptic seizures. Epilepsia 26:303–309

Dahl JA, Melin L, Lund L (1987) Effects of a contingent relaxation treatment programme on adults with refractory epileptic seizures. Epilepsia 28:125–132

Deyo RA, Diehl AK, Rosenthal M (1986) How many days of bed rest for acute low back pain? N Engl J Med 315:1064–1070

Engel BT (1986) Psychosomatic medicine, behavioral medicine, just plain medicine. Psychosom Med 48:466–478
Hogarty GE, Goldberg SC, The Collaborative Study Group (1973) Drug and sociotherapy in the aftercare of the schizophrenic patients: one-year relapse rates. Arch Gen Psychiatry 28:54–64
Holder HD, Hallan JB (1981) Medical care and alcoholism treatment costs and utilization: a five-year analysis of the California pilot project to provide health insurance coverage for alcoholism. Mimeographed report for the National Institute on Alcohol Abuse and Alcoholism
Laudenschlager ML, Ryan SM, Drugan RC, Hysow RL, Maier SF (1983) Coping and immunosuppression: inescapable but not escapable shock suppresses lymphocyte proliferation. Science 221:568–570
Leitenberg H (1976) Handbook of behavior modification and behavior therapy. Prentice-Hall, Englewood Cliffs, NJ
Linton SJ (1985) The relationship between activity and chronic back pain. Pain 21:289–294
Linton SJ, Götestam KG (1984) A controlled study of the effects of applied relaxation and applied relaxation plus operant procedures in the regulation of chronic pain. Br J Clin Psychol 23:291–299
Linton SJ, Götestam KG (1985) Controlling pain reports through operant conditioning: a laboratory demonstration. Percept Mot Skills 60:427–437
Lovibond SH, Birrell PC, Langeludecke P (1986) Changing coronary heart disease risk-factor status: the effects of three behavioral programs. J Behav Med 9:415–437
Maguire P, Pentol A, Allen D, Tait A, Brooke M, Sellwood R (1982) Cost of counselling women who undergo mastectomy. Br Med J 284:1933–1935
Marlatt A, Gordon J (1985) Relapse prevention: maintenance strategies in addictive behavior change. Guilford, New York
Melamed BG, Siegel LJ (1980) Behavioral medicine, practical applications in health care. Springer, New York
Melin L, Götestam KG (1980) A behavioral approach to drug abuse. Drug Alcohol Depend 5:5–25
Metal'nikov S, Chorine V (1926) Rôle des réflexes conditionnels dans la formation des anticorps. C R Soc Bio 99:142
Nachemson A (1985) Work for all: for those with low back pain as well. Clin Orthop 179:77–85
Puska P (1973) The North Karelia project: an attempt at community prevention of cardiovascular disease. WHO Chron 27:55–58
Puska P, Tuomilehto J, Salonen J, Nissinen A, Virtamo J et al. (1983) The North Karelia project: evaluation of a comprehensive programme for control of cardiovascular diseases in 1972–77 in North Karelia, Finland. WHO Monograph, Geneva
Roccella EJ et al. (1986) Non-pharmacological approaches to the control of high blood pressure. Hypertension 8:444–467
Saylor KE (1987) Enhancing a videocasette weight loss program through self-directed adherence training. Doctoral thesis, Stanford University School of Education, Stanford, California
Schwartz JL (1987) Review and evaluation of smoking cessation methods. US Department of Health and Human Services, National Institutes of Health (Publ No 87-2940), Washington, D.C., Government Printing Office
Smith GR, Monson RA, Ray DC (1986) Psychiatric consultation in somatization disorder: a randomized controlled study. N Engl J Med 314:1407–1413
Sternbach R (1974) Pain patients: traits and treatment. Academic Press, London
Suls J, Sanders GS, Labrecque MS (1986) Attempting to control blood pressure without systematic instruction: when advice is counterproductive. J Behav Med 9:567–577
Ulrich RS (1984) View through a window may influence recovery from surgery. Science 224:420–421
Yates A (1980) Biofeedback and the modification of behavior. Plenum Press, New York

Behavioral Aspects of Physical Illness in Children and Adolescents

E. A. Sand

Introduction

In the field of child psychiatry and child mental health, specific elements such as behavioral symptoms have to be considered in the complex and subtle network of interactions between physical-somatic and psychiatric factors.

One may assume that due to the plasticity of the young brain (Levin et al. 1983) at the early stages of its development (the fetal and neonatal periods), the prognosis of certain types of lesions is more favorable than in adults. However, this may be only partly true. On the other hand, the anatomical growth of the neurological structures, as well as their functional development from the early fetal stages onwards may be influenced by environmental factors, as much in a positive as in a negative sense (e.g., through viral infection or through ionizing radiations). Account must also be taken of the occurrence of optimal moments or periods when, as Spitz (1958) has pointed out, new stages of developmental progress may be achieved in an optimal way and, often, quickly. Conversely, if such optimal opportunities are not used, the long-term consequences may be negative, e.g., in situations of early deprivation (Ainsworth 1962; Bowlby 1951; Fischer and Berger 1987), though evaluation of the long-term outcome of such early environmental influences is methodologically difficult (Sand 1984). In these interactions, the role of the immediate social environment (mother, father, siblings) as well as of the wider environment (age-peers, school) should not be underestimated.

Analyses of this problem are carried out on various assumptions, which depend on the scientific orientation (clinical, epidemiological, neurobiological, interdisciplinary) of the research team. In some projects, behavioral symptomatology is used as a starting point, leading to inferences about pathogenic mechanisms. In others, the successive steps, from possible causal factors to the clinical outcome, are considered in a more logical, i.e., chronological order.

Some examples of this latter type of study will be presented first because of their theoretical interest. However, behavioral symptoms also deserve attention, since more often than not, clinicians are obliged to carry out the difficult task of elaborating causal hypotheses retrospectively.

Ecole de Santé Publique de l'Université Libre de Bruxelles, Campus Erasme 595, Route de Lennik, 808, B-1070 Bruxelles

Interaction Between Mental and Physical Illness
Edited by R. Öhman et al.

Genetic and Intrauterine Variables

In the field of genetics and genetic epidemiology, a great variety of neurological and behavioral syndromes have been described. Recently, new data with significant results in the field of genetic epidemiology have been presented concerning schizophrenia, generalized seizures (King et al. 1984), affective disorders (Mendlewicz et al. 1987), and infantile autism (Sanua 1986 a, b). Mednick and Kandel (1987) indicate that viral or physical agents, acting on the brain tissue between the third and sixth months of pregnancy, are associated with a significant increase in the incidence of childhood autism. They also point out the possible effects of interactions between genetic or congenital influences and early childhood life events, such as family disruption.

Because of their preventive implications, the complications of pregnancy have been repeatedly analysed. A recent study from the Dundee Developmental Screening Programme, has been published by Taylor et al. (1985). Severe cases of neurological and mental disabilities were rare, though previous studies had shown that 13%–16% of all preschool children have a neurodevelopmental disability. This study analysed 300 children with primary disability, including mental retardation (25), global delay (52), cerebral palsy (12), motor delay (50), speech delay (91), and behavior disorder (49).

While the social class (or more accurately, the socioeconomic level) of the family is linked significantly to most of the above disorders, it yields only partial explanations of them. Complications of pregnancy such as severe hypertension, antepartum hemorrhage and preterm uterine activity are associated with one or several of these disorders, with the exception of cerebral palsy, which has an association with fetal tachycardia occurring during labor.

In 1963, Gruenwald had indicated the impact on various organs of the condition of smallness for gestational age in babies, but the brain is not as affected by it, in terms of weight reduction, as are other organs, e.g., the liver or spleen. This author underlined the greater vulnerability of the brain tissue during the later stages of fetal development, though others, like Mednick (personal communication), emphasize a greater vulnerability during the second trimester of pregnancy. While low birth-weight and prematurity (short gestation) are considered as risk factors, particularly in relation to cerebral palsy, these factors are not associated with seizure disorders (Ellenberg and Nelson 1979). Other authors (e.g., Saint-Anne Dargassies 1977) hold that though motor impairments may be present, psychological, behavioral and intellectual impairments are more frequent in children who were born premature or were small for gestational age.

In 1982, Walther and Ramaekers published a long-term follow-up study of 25 full-term infants classified as having experienced subacute fetal distress and 25 controls; the distress was "most probably related to intra-uterine malnutrition." Screening was carried out at 3 years by use of a behavior screening questionnaire (BSQ), a behavior observation report (BOR), and a neurological assessment (NA). Significant differences appeared between the index cases and the control group in various behavioral and neurological fields: fears (BSQ & BOR); activity and concentration (BOR); posture, standing (NA); speed, smoothness and adequacy of motility (NA); and dyskinesia or choreiform movements (NA).

Neonatal Pathology

While the plasticity of the young brain might reduce the probability of occurrence of later somatic or psychiatric pathology (Levin et al. 1983), a number of studies indicate that children who have suffered damage to their central nervous system later present significantly higher proportions of psychomotor retardation and of neurological and behavioral disturbances than do other children.

Baran's follow-up study (Baran et al. 1982) of 252 Polish newborn children, which included variables such as maternal health, the course of pregnancy and labor, and the neonatal and infant health of the child, confirms earlier evaluations carried out in France (Saint-Anne Dargassies 1977) and in the United States (Ellenberg and Nelson 1979). These observations all underline the important functions of preventive action and correct care during pregnancy, labor, and early infancy, as well as the responsibility for this of the health care system, including the technical and organizational components of obstetric and neonatal care.

However, recent research (Paneth et al. 1981) points to an increase in the frequency of cerebral palsy between 1960 and 1970, though not as marked as the previous decrease between 1950 and 1960. This phenomenon should probably be attributed to the interaction between a reduction in the neonatal death rate and an increase in that of neurological impairment; both could be linked to the quality of intensive neonatal care. Indeed, cases of severe mental retardation were observed eight times more frequently in very low birth-weight babies (survivors), compared with normal birth-weight children.

Though the conclusions of this particular research might be based on "unduly pessimistic" assumptions, the effects of the decline in mortality of very low birth-weight newborns could result in increased prevalence rates of impairment. The effects will be beneficial "only if the impairment rate among low birth-weight survivors declines more rapidly than does their neonatal mortality rate" (Paneth et al. 1981). This is clearly an open question, which deserves more investigation, not only by those in the field of neonatal care, but also from other perspectives.

Postnatal Neurological Disorders and Behavioral Symptoms

Associations between neurological disorders and behavioral or psychiatric disorders were mentioned in the medical literature as early as 1854 by Falret, and some decades ago by Kanner (1957).

Epidemiological Aspects

An important proportion of the published observations are based on clinical samples recruited in hospital services or in extramural consultations. This means that the observed rates refer mainly to those categories of children whose behavioral disorders are severe enough to justify regular and specialized medical care.

Conversely, one might assume that other children who have also suffered from neurological disorders either do not present any behavioral problems later on or, if they do present such symptoms, these are not perceived as serious enough, in the view of the parents or educators, to justify medical or psychological care. Some authors, e.g., de Barbot (1984), consider that there is no statistical evidence that children suffering from cerebral motor abnormalities (*infirmes moteurs cérébraux*) present more or less behavior disorders than other children.

Moreover, there may be a risk, as Kalra et al. (1982) state of ignoring altogether the psychiatric and behavioral components of organic lesions of the central nervous system. These authors presented data from a clinical sample ($n = 70$) of 5- to 12-year-old children, investigated in the Department of Pediatrics of the Medical College of Agra. The pathologies considered were sequelae of epilepsy, encephalitis, and meningitis, but no details are given within these broad categories of diseases. The most highly prevalent observed disorders were: hyperactivity (42.9%), aggressiveness (32.9%), obstinacy (27.1%), irritability (22.9%), temper tantrums (21.5%), and emotional lability (21.5%); speech defects were observed in 10%. While the prevalence of these symptoms might differ somewhat from one CNS disorder to another, the most frequent behavioral problems were observed throughout all the CNS disorders, though irritability seemed to be more frequent in the sequelae of meningitis.

In this field of clinical investigation, special mention should be made of the general lack of knowledge about the early behavioral symptomatology of cerebral disorders. The symptoms may be misleading and of low specificity, and their significance may be ignored for long periods (Basquin 1982).

Daléry et al. (1981) from a study of a small clinical sample, indicated the possible diagnostic pitfalls which may prevent clinicians from correctly recognizing the neuroorganic nature of psychological disturbances in children. These may constitute the first, and possibly for longer periods the only symptoms of organic disease.

Some Postnatal Causal Hypotheses and Mechanisms

Possible causal factors are manifold, but three main categories are mentioned frequently in the literature. The first, which is more than ever a priority now through the recent increase in incidence of herpetic infections and of AIDS, relates to infectious syndromes, such as meningitis and encephalitis. Moreover, recent publications point to the role that an almost forgotten disease – encephalitis lethargica – could still be playing (Espir and Spalding 1956; Greenough and Davis 1983). The relationships, in this case between CNS lesions and behavioral symptoms, are well known.

The second category includes both benign and malignant brain tumors of various types: the occurrence of psychological symptoms in some types, e.g., supra-sellar, had been mentioned in 1934 by the Belgian neurologists Van Bogaert and Martin.

The third category of causal factors is that of head injuries, which compared with the other causes probably is associated with a lower risk of ignoring or underestimating the origin of the ensuing psychological and behavioral disorders. Yet, although this is a fairly well-explored field of child neurology and psychiatry, and an extensive study had already been published in 1936 by Blau, nevertheless many aspects of the consequences of head injuries are as yet not well known.

The book edited by Shapiro (1983) contains a rich quantity of research data, the chapter by Levin et al. (1983) giving information on closed head injuries (CHI) – mainly on their early neurological symptoms and long-term sequelae. However, the concept of plasticity of the young brain is clearly not applicable to all kinds of lesions: if children seem to recover better than adults from focal lesions, "there is no impressive evidence indicating that immaturity confers any advantage in withstanding the effects of diffuse cerebral insult." Is this plasticity a myth or a fact? Indeed, the main support for the plasticity concept, stems from follow-up studies of language development after localized lesions of the left hemisphere (Levin et al. 1983). This area deserves more attention and research.

On the other hand, the residual psychological and psychosocial effects have not been explored sufficiently. It is often very difficult to make a clear distinction between premorbid behavior disorders, possibly reinforced by the CHI, and the behavioral consequences of the head injury. However, the conclusions of the research are contradictory, since both premorbid influences and that of the injury seem to be important.

There is more clarity with respect to psychological functions after CHI: while memory and psychomotor abilities are more severely affected, "language development is relatively resistent to the effects of CHI" (Levin et al. 1983). Finally, the epileptic syndrome and its behavioral consequences also need to be considered.

Examples of Psychological and Behavioral Consequences

In this field, a great richness of information is available, particularly from the book *Brain-Behavior Relationship* (Merikangas 1981). All over the world, aggressiveness and violence in youth have become a problem of serious concern, not only for parents and educators, but also for public health authorities, police, criminal courts, social scientists, etc. On the other hand, it appears that from early childhood onwards, symptoms of aggressive behavior are, more than others, stable in time and significantly associated with various other behavior disorders (Bronson 1966; Sand 1972).

Merikangas has thrown new light on an ancient controversy between sociological and neurobiological hypotheses on the genesis of violent behavior, distinguishing different types of violent behavior in the human species. The main problem is not the violent reaction to specific stimuli – which may be explained by psychosocial factors – but the response which is "apparently spontaneous or which occurs without a clear stimulus-response relationship." The need is stressed to analyse in all cases (but especially in children and adolescents, because of the social, educational, and developmental components involved), a wide set of elements, such as "mood, movement, sensation, cognition and consciousness." In this analysis, roles of six components are considered, from the stimulus and the stimulus threshold to the fixed action pattern and the nature of the response inhibition. Merikangas emphasizes that fairly specific neurological disorders are observed in many cases of aggressive behavior, though this conclusion does not contradict the importance of economic and psychosocial factors, e.g., living conditions, social and economic inequities.

The work of Mednick and Kandel (1987) points to the joint influence of both these categories of components. They have observed the interaction between specific kinds of physical anomalies and of social influences, such as family stability vs lack of stability: violent behavior was significantly more frequent in adolescents presenting jointly a high level of minor physical anomalies and a high level of family instability.

In addition to aggressive-behavior symptoms, the neurological aspects of perceptual, motor, and attentional deficits in children must not be forgotten. This was pointed out by Rasmussen et al. (1983), whose survey in Sweden was based on a representative sample of 6-year-old Swedish schoolchildren. One aim was to describe the "neurological deviations of children suffering from minimal brain damage (MBD)." From a sample, of 3448 children, 141 with symptoms of attention deficit were selected for more complete assessment, based on a questionnaire completed by preschool teachers. In this cross-sectional description, significant differences were found between these 141 children and a control group: speech and language deficits ($p<0.001$), muscular tone and reflexes ($p<0.001$), oculomotor dysfunction ($p<0.01$), tremor ($p<0.001$), and left-handedness ($p<0.05$). Eight children, all of whom had suffered MBD, were described as having psychotic behavior.

This study raises important questions about the meaning and both short- and long-term consequences of these symptoms in MBD children. Compared with such optimal representative samples, the conclusions of follow-up studies carried out on hospital samples may not be generalized. Indeed, they may induce a seriously biased image of the future of these children, whether in the area of motor performance or in relation to school success and failure.

Behavioral Aspects and Consequences of Somatic Illness

As far as diabetic children are concerned, the literature contains only a few comprehensive studies, in terms of sampling and of the number of symptoms considered jointly. A study in Sweden by Ahnsjö et al. (1981) presents interesting data which are in contrast with earlier studies and their somewhat contradictory results. It was based on a geographically representative sample in Stockholm recruited from hospitals, and completed by a matched control-group ($n=60$; age, 4–17 years). The research tools used were: a mental state protocol, prepared by the hospital psychiatrist; an evaluation of the social situation of the family; the Terman-Merrill test and the Rorschach test. The authors concluded that on the whole, there were no clear differences in the mental states of these children: the most conspicuous observation was the normal behavior of the diabetic children and their families. Nor were there any significant differences in intellectual capacity between the diabetic children and the control group.

However, at onset of the disease, the diabetic children showed an increased level of anxiety, which diminished later, according to Rorschach results. The level of tolerance of anxiety was not lower in the diabetic children, but they showed a "greater vulnerability" in the Rorschach test, and were also more depressed. However, their level of maturity was increased beyond expectation.

It was concluded that the quality and strictness of the care given the children "might even have a supportive effect." In the same sense, Hoare (1984), studying dependency in diabetic and epileptic children, could not find any inappropriate dependency in his sample of diabetics. But conversely, inappropriate dependency was found in the epileptic children, who also showed a significant increase of psychiatric disturbance, possibly due to their dependency.

Another topic in this field is the problem of the psychological, behavioral and social consequences of "demanding clinical trials." A study by Kinmonth et al. (1983), undertaken within the framework of research on the effects of two contrasting diets on diabetic control, was carried out on a small sample of 11- to 17-year-old children. It showed very clearly that in spite of the care given to the selection of the sample and the consent of the children and their parents, these children "will have social and emotional problems." Hence, "prevision for the necessary (emotional) support should be built into the design of such trials."

Conclusions

While some of the areas considered above are fairly well covered by research, more often there is an impression of lack of knowledge, mainly due to the multivariate character of the problems, as well as to an apparent lack of action in the field of child psychiatry, compared with adult psychiatry. However, there is one specific area which is quite well covered: the physical and psychological development of children. For example, social interaction both in family and in institutions, has been and is being subject to adequate study.

But the interaction between neurophysiological versus social and psychological variables deserves more attention. Indeed, the behavioral problems of children suffering from CNS disorders raise the problem of their education and care. The development of subtle interactions between somatic and psychological factors can be observed both in the child's behavior and in the reactions of parents and educators. The management of these reactions, for the ultimate benefit of the child and of the whole family-system, requires a broad perception of the neurobiological pathology, as well as of the emotional and relational interactions. The way the child itself feels that it is regarded, looked at, loved, or possibly rejected, should be carefully considered.

The main areas to be considered more carefully, in the light of the available literature, can be summarized as follows:

- Pregnancy complications: type of complications and factors (including alcohol- and drug-related problems); analysis of confounding variables
- Early diagnosis of fetal distress: required measures and care, evaluation of care
- Health-care management for newborns, i.e., low birth-weight babies; need for follow-up studies
- Neurological disorders and their consequences: prevalence, specificity, early symptoms, neurological symptoms, and reactions of the social environment
- Early stages of brain tumors: symptoms, evolution
- Head injury (e.g., closed injury): lack of indices of acute stages (coma scale); links between the original lesion(s) and later symptomatology; the plasticity of the young brain, its limits, the overall fields of application and validity of the concept
- Minimal brain dysfunction (MBD): prospective investigations
- Aggressiveness: interaction between neurobiological and psychosocial factors; classifications of aggressive behavior, in relation to social versus somatic factors
- Health care management research: who should take care of patients with MBD, with various types of aggressive behavior, etc.?
- How should personnel be trained to acquire the needed skills and attitudes to cope with the particular, multifactorial situations described in this chapter?

References

Ahnsjö S, Humble K, Larsson Y et al. (1981) Personality changes and social adjustment during the first three years of diabetes in children. Acta Paediatr Scand 70:321–327

Ainsworth B (1962) The effects of maternal deprivation: a review of findings and controversy in the context of research strategy. In: Deprivation of maternal care. WHO, Geneva (Public health papers, no 14)

Baran J, Kulmaga T, Losiowski Z, Zardecka T (1982) Psychomotor development in children with neonatal period pathology in the first two years of life. Pediatr Pol 57:95–100
Basquin M (1982) Les débuts psychiques des affections cérébrales chez l'enfant. Entretiens de Bichat. Expansion Scientif. Française, Paris, pp 321–324
Blau A (1936) Mental changes following head trauma in children. Arch Neurol Psychiatr 35:723–769
Bowlby J (1951) Soins maternels et santé mentale. WHO, Geneva (sér monogr 2)
Bronson W (1966) Central orientations: a study of behavior organization from childhood to adolescence. Child Dev 37:125–155
Daléry J, Boucand MH, Maillet J et al. (1981) Tumeurs cérébrales et malformations vasculaires à masque psychiatrique chez l'enfant. A propos d'une expérience personnelle. Neuropsychiatr Enfance 29(11–12):625–630
de Barbot F (1984) Le sens des troubles du comportement chez les IMC. Motricité cérébrale 5:41–47
Ellenberg JH, Nelson KB (1979) Birth weight and gestational age in children with cerebral palsy or seizure disorders. Am J Dis Child 133:1044–1048
Espir MLE, Spalding JMK (1956) Three recent cases of encephalitis lethargica. Br Med J [Clin Res] I:1141–1144
Falret J (1854) Mémoire sur la folie circulaire. Bull Acad Méd Paris 19:382–400
Fischer G, Berger M (1987)Sind seelische Verletzungen in der frühen Kindheit unbedenklich? Der Kinderarzt 18(5):639–646
Greenough A, Davis JA (1983) Encephalitis lethargica: mystery of the past or undiagnosed disease of the present? Lancet I(8330):922–923
Gruenwald P (1963) Chronic fetal distress and placental insufficiency. Biol Neonate 5:215–265
Hoare P (1984) Does illness foster dependency? Study of epileptic and diabetic children. Dev Med Child Neurol 26(1):20–24
Kalra A, Agarval V, Misra N et al. (1982) Analysis of psychiatric symptoms in neurological disorders in children. Arch Child Health (Calcutta) 24(2):40–45
Kanner L (1957) Child psychiatry, 3rd edn. Thomas, Springfield
King MC, Lee GM, Spinner NB et al. (1984) Genetic epidemiology. Annu Rev Public Health 5:1–52
Kinmonth AL, Lindsay MKM, Baum JD (1983) Social and emotional complications in a clinical trial among adolescents with diabetes mellitus. Br Med J [Clin Res] 286:952–954
Levin HS, Eisenberg HM, Miner ME (1983) Neuropsychologic findings in head injured children (chap 9). In: Shapiro K (ed) Pediatric head trauma. Futura, Mount Kisco, pp 223–240
Mednick SA, Kandel E (1987) Genetic and perinatal factors in violence. In: Mednick SA, Kandel E (ed) Biological contributions to crime causation. Nijhoff, The Hague
Mendlewicz J, Simon P, Sevy S et al. (1987) Polymorphic DNA marker on X chromosome and manic depression. Lancet i(8544):1230–1231
Merikangas JR (1981) The neurology of violence. In: Merikangas JR (ed) Brain-behaviour relationship. Lexington, Toronto, pp 155–185
Paneth N, Kiely JI, Stein Z, Susser M (1981) Cerebral palsy and newborn care III: estimated prevalence of cerebral palsy under different rates of mortality and impairment of low birth-weight infants. Dev Med Child Neurol 23:801–807
Rasmussen P, Gillberg C, Waldenström E, Svenson B (1983) Perceptual, motor and attentional deficits in seven-year-old children: neurological and neurodevelopmental aspects. Dev Med Child Neurol 25:315–333
Saint-Anne Dargassies S (1977) Long-term neurological follow-up study of 286 truly premature infants I: neurological sequelae. Dev Med Child Neurol 19:462–478
Sand EA (1972) Symptômes de comportement d'enfants belges observés par leurs mères: I. Stabilité de 3 à 9 ans, II. Associations entre symptômes. Rev Neuropsychiatr Infant Hyg Ment Enfance 20(3–4):239–251, 253–265

Sand EA (1984) Ontogeny of bonding-attachment: epidemiological and public health aspects. Prog Reprod Biol Med 11:69–73
Sanua V (1986a) Letter to the editor: the organic etiology of infantile autism, a critical review of the literature. Int J Neurosci 30:195–225
Sanua V (1986b) A comparative study of opinions of USA and European professionals on the etiology of infantile autism. Int J Soc Psychiatry 32(2):16–29
Shapiro K (ed) (1983) Pediatric head trauma. Futura, Mount Kisco
Spitz RA (1958) La première année de la vie de l'enfant. Presses Univ de France, Paris
Taylor DJ, Howie PW, Davidson J et al. (1985) Do pregnancy complications contribute to neurodevelopmental disability? Lancet i(8431):713–718
Van Bogaert L, Martin P (1934) Tumeur supra-sellaire avec symptomatologie psychique. Groupement belge d'étude oto-rhino-ophthalmologique et neuro-chirurgicale, 24 November 1934, Daléry
Walther FJW, Ramaekers LHJ (1982) Developmental aspects of subacute fetal distress: behaviour problems and neurological dysfunction. Early Hum Dev 6:1–10

Summaries of Discussion

H. L. Freeman

AIDS

From the beginning, the problem of AIDS has been associated with preexisting handicap (homosexuality, drug use, imprisonment, hemophilia), involving psychosocial stress, such as prejudice or isolation. So far, research has not dealt with the psychosocial or psychosomatic aspects of AIDS – for instance, there has been no comparison between coping mechanisms in hemophiliacs and homosexuals. In the case of homosexuals and drug addicts, research needs to be concerned particularly with how their behavior can be changed by education and advice. This seems to be particularly difficult for addicts. Comparisons could be made with coping behavior in other chronic or life-threatening conditions.

Another problem is how to reduce risk-taking behavior in heterosexuals who have multiple partners, particularly when there may be an impact on spouses and families. Young people use condoms in an entirely different way from older, more established couples; they have a general tendency to deny risks. It is not known why certain seropositive persons do not develop AIDS, but it is possible that psychological factors influence this, or influence the course of the disease. More research is needed on psychological aspects of immunology – for instance, effects of anxiety or depression – or changes produced by conditioning; more should also be known about coping strategies and risk-taking behavior. Greenland, which has culturally determined promiscuity, would be an ideal natural laboratory for research of all kinds, including evaluating interventions.

Little is known about education of the general population, but a recent national campaign in the UK ('Don't Die of Ignorance') was almost certainly quite ineffective. There has been little evaluation of educational techniques. More needs to be known about the early clinical manifestations of AIDS, and particularly about neuropsychological symptoms, such as fatigue and poor memory. There is a problem of aggressive behavior by some infected individuals, and health personnel need better advice and training, based on more ac-

The Royal College of Psychiatrists, 17 Belgrave Square, London SWIX 8PG

Interaction Between Mental and Physical Illness
Edited by R. Öhman et al.

curate information. Methadone programs may need to be developed, though in the USA, they are no longer regarded as very effective.

Since resources are limited, it may be better to concentrate on established public health methods and clinical care – screening, contact tracing, isolation of infected cases – but this is not being done. The ethical issues are no different from those of fatal infections in the past, and AIDS is no worse than TB or smallpox was, before these were overcome. There has been little discussion of the way that diagnosis or control is being hampered, at present, by legalistic restrictions.

Epilepsy

Psychiatrists generally show a lack of interest in epilepsy, though the important scientific questions about it are now just beginning to be appropriate to the level of scientific knowledge that we possess. It represents one of the most promising avenues for correlating brain function with specific types of psychopathology. The basis of any progress will be thorough clinical study of individual cases, particularly of temporal-lobe epilepsy – as Hughlings Jackson predicted, a century ago. Epilepsy is common, affecting 5%–10% of the population at some point, but most of these people have no psychiatric problems.

Complex partial seizures are of particular interest to psychiatry, and may not involve the motor system. They may involve disturbance of consciousness, of thought, of affect, or of behavior – but these disturbances are not necessarily ictal. The broad spectrum of psychopathology which is found in the major psychoses is also found in epilepsy, and suicide is one of the forms of abnormal behavior which occurs. There is an interictal behavior syndrome, which has three main forms: first, changed sexual behavior; second, religious or esoteric preoccupation; and third, hypergraphia, which is also found in chronic schizophrenia, and might be a mechanism for coping with temporal lobe dysfunction.

Studies of the localization of temporal foci have produced contradictory results, but there is an excess of left-handedness among epileptics, particularly those with psychoses. Some patients diagnosed as epileptic are actually found to have schizophrenia or neurosis, when they are investigated more fully, but putting them on long-term anticonvulsant medication may have harmful results. Much more cooperation is needed between psychiatrists and neurologists to improve the quality of diagnosis.

There is a definite association between schizophrenia and temporal lobe epilepsy, but it is not clear how limbic function is related to this. Possibly, it generates emotional overinvolvement. It is not clear how much psychopathology in epileptics is related to structural changes, and how much to abnormal levels of brain activity. Temporal-lobe epilepsy may also be related to the activity of other regions of the brain such as the frontal lobes, but the temporal lobes act as the 'gates' to these regions.

Since the vulnerability to strong stimuli is found both in epilepsy and in schizophrenia, a retreat into fantasy or immobility might be a coping response to either condition.

Physical Morbidity and Mortality

There are very consistent findings of excess mortality among psychiatric patients, particularly those resident in mental hospitals. This involves all causes of death – natural and unnatural – except malignant neoplasms. It seems to be nonspecific. It is possible that neuroleptics have an antitumor effect. The risk is higher in younger patients, and at the beginning of illness, in the first year of hospital stay. In schizophrenia, the risk is very high at first, but approaches that of the general population, as time goes on.

The mortality of schizophrenia has not changed recently, but that of affective disorder has declined. There are differing trends from other diagnostic categories, and results are affected by many selective and intervening variables. Violent causes of death have become more important in recent years, and are related to psychoses.

As far as depression is concerned, mortality might be seen as the final common path of a number of processes. Good mental health is a powerful protective factor against premature death.

In research, there are methodological problems of collecting an adequate sample size, doing multicenter studies, determining causes of death, and using multiaxial diagnostic systems.

Further research is needed to understand contradictory results in relation to cancer and cardiovascular disease, and to investigate the relationship of immune processes to psychopathology (a topic which is also relevant to AIDS). The design of studies relating to immunology is likely to be very difficult.

Well-controlled prospective studies among large, representative populations of psychiatric patients would be useful, taking into account selection mechanisms, preexisting diseases, effects of abnormal behavior, and variables related to treatment and lifestyles.

Psychological Contributions to Physical Illness

Research is not just adding to knowledge, but helping professionals to answer questions (from government or the public), and providing the means to bring about change. The data produced by research are essential for teaching and in advising how health services should be provided.

Treatment, which can improve impaired function, is different from *management*, which improves the social situation and emotional independence of those who suffer handicap. The present methods of delivering health care, particularly for those who have long-term problems, are very complex and expensive. Could this be done more simply, but more effectively?

Existing theories (such as personality types, life-events, or stress-coping mechanisms) may no longer be stimulating for research. New ones should embrace both biological and sociological aspects. For instance, why do only *some* people adopt a sick role – why do the majority not do so? New multiaxial, problem-orientated classification systems may need to be developed. Those used by research workers may be different from those used by clinicians, who have to give information to patients. A simple scale with social, physical, and psychological dimensions (in which only the psychological and social are correlated), might be of value in chronic disorders.

How can behavior be changed, e.g., so that irresponsible driving – a major cause of mortality – is controlled? Known risk factors, e.g., alcohol consumption and smoking, are not being confronted in most countries. Why not? Decisions by most governments bear no relationship to research findings.

Though acute services are usually good, long-term care in most countries is very poor, e.g., for the brain-injured who are not so uncommon and who may live for very many years. How can self-help be encouraged, and carers (usually relatives) be supported better?

Psychiatric Consequences of High Technology in Medical Care

By definition, methods employing high technology are of restricted availability, and access to them involves some form of rationing, whether implicit or explicit. Even if there was unlimited equipment, there would not be enough skilled staff to operate it. One objective is safer and less invasive investigation, and it is assumed that if all conditions were detected earlier, outcome would be improved – but this is not necessarily the case.

As well as investigation, high technology also involves treatment settings – intensive care, transplantation, total parenteral nutrition, neurosurgery, radiotherapy – and there is a danger that the elaboration of equipment and monitoring procedures will result in little personal contact between the staff and patients. There is a danger of substituting technicians for caring staff.

In renal dialysis, about half the patients experience significant depression, and about one-third have marked anxiety; their level of distress is similar to that of psychiatric patients. Needed areas of research include better tools of assessment, prospective and multicenter studies, and measurements of the quality of life.

There are ethical issues which remain to be explored, and problems affecting the staff in these units might be helped by better training and by Balint groups – though this has not been generally accepted. Balint groups of surgeons is a fascinating idea.

The use of high-technology methods may sometimes involve impossible choices for patients and their families – 'playing for the whole box.' The denial mechanism may in fact be essential if patients and families are to cope with these situations. We need to know when and why it fails, and what is the role of family support in general.

Doctors may also practice denial, perhaps in the form of overoptimism. 'High-tech' solutions tend to be introduced before they have ever been properly evaluated, and may need more cost-benefit studies. How much of them can or should any economy afford? There is much interest in alternatives, such as hospices for the dying, which may be cheaper. Only certain types of staff are suitable for work in high-tech units, and most will not remain in them long.

There is a major difficulty in the low rate of referral of these patients for psychiatric help. How can the rate of referral be increased? How can staff become more patient-centered? and more aware of the emotional aspects of these situations? Although negative aspects are emphasized, some patients do find these units comforting, when they have life-threatening conditions. It would be useful to have an assessment package which nurses could readily give, to assess patients' emotional state and degree of confusion. There are particular implications for children, and those born with the aid of high-technology obstetrics ought to be followed up over long periods.

Implications for Future Research

H. L. FREEMAN

The purpose of this symposium was primarily to determine the most needed areas of research concerning the relationship of psychiatric and physical disorder. These needs can be summarized under a number of headings, related to the papers and discussions which appear earlier in the present volume.

With regard to the clinical aspects of the psychiatric consequences of physical illness, possible lines of research include the following:

- Clinical study of the asthenic-depressive syndrome, including determination of whether or not it has a neurobiological basis
- Examination of the way in which mental states influence physical disorders, such as ischemic heart disease, including possible biochemical mechanisms
- Development of psychological methods which could be shown to promote the healing of physical disorders
- Development of teaching programs for nonpsychiatric doctors and health professionals, with evaluation of these programs
- Improvement of methods for early recognition of minimal cerebral dysfunction
- Precise definition of brain lesions that correspond to clinical phenomena, through the use of new imaging methods
- Prospective studies to determine the psychological consequences of accidental injuries
- Determination of any family factors that are related to psychiatric symptoms which result from a given level of stress

In relation to questions of physical morbidity and mortality in psychiatric patients, four principal areas of research have been proposed: First, an attempt should be made to reduce the methodological problems which have been a barrier to progress, e.g., sample size, the complexities of multicenter studies, and the use of multiaxial diagnostic systems in determining causes of death. Second, an attempt should be made to resolve the hitherto contradictory results which have emerged regarding cancer and cardiovascular disease in psychiatric patients. Third, the relationship between immune processes and psychopathology, as illustrated by AIDS, should be examined. Fourth, prospective

The Royal College of Psychiatrists, 17 Belgrave Square, London SWIX 8PG

Interaction Between Mental and Physical Illness
Edited by R. Öhman et al.

studies of large and representative populations of psychiatric patients should be developed to determine their experience of morbidity and mortality.

Knowledge of neurobiological aspects of the psychiatric consequences of physical illness will most likely progress along six suggested primary areas of research:

- Application of recent knowledge to the study of mind-body interactions
- Possible role of glutamate antagonists in the negative symptoms of schizophrenia
- Study of antagonists causing disturbance of brain function, in contrast with the usual study of agonists
- Extension of the use of new imaging methods (e.g., PET) to investigate the action of dopamine in the brain
- Examination of the role of peptides in immune modulation to help elucidate the interaction of physical illness and psychosocial states
- Search for situations where effective treatments overlap, in terms of brain mechanisms, since most basic psychotropic drugs have been discovered by accident

Further research on the psychiatric aspects of AIDS was proposed along the following directions:

- Evaluation of the educational methods now being used for the general public, high-risk groups, and young people
- Examination of the effect of psychological factors on immunological processes
- Investigation of the coping strategies used, e.g., by seropositive cases, and comparison of these with the strategies used in other disorders
- Improvement of the clinical study of early neuropsychological manifestations of AIDS
- Finding ways of improving staff education and training in the management of AIDS
- Determination as to whether established public health techniques can be used in effective ways for AIDS, perhaps in relation to one community, which could act as a 'population laboratory'

In relation to the use of high-technology techniques in medicine, it was proposed that research should be concerned in the first place with evaluation of their use and comparison of them with alternatives. Second, the important question was raised of how the rate of referral to psychiatric diagnosis and care of patients receiving these techniques could be increased. Third, was the question whether simple instruments can be devised to assess the psychiatric state of patients in this situation. Fourth, a need was expressed for prospective studies to determine the long-term effects on children involved with the use of high-technology procedures. Fifth, it was recommended that the roles be examined of family support for such patients and of the process of denial – by doctors, relatives, and the patients themselves. Sixth, better methods of staff training, such as perhaps Balint-type seminars, were called for. Finally, it was emphasized that there is a need to know what quality of life is experienced by patients when high-technology techniques are used to treat them.

With regard to research into the behavioral aspects of physical illness, it was submitted that this should follow five directions:

- Evaluation of psychosocial interventions
- Investigation of how coping strategies develop in patients and relatives
- Comparative studies of different treatment approaches to a problem
- Assessment of the effect of financial policies, such as disability pensions
- The cost-benefit studies of different methods of the management of chronic diseases, with the benefits assessed mainly in terms of patients' quality of life

In the case of epilepsy, numerous lines of research were proposed concerning the relationship between this disease and psychiatric disturbances:

- Defining better questions, e.g., what are the psychological manifestations of temporal-lobe dysfunction?
- Carrying out more detailed clinical studies, particularly of temporal-lobe epilepsy, as the basis for defining syndromes; in these studies, better behavioral measurements are required
- Undertaking large epidemiological community studies, e.g., of the relationship between epilepsy and psychopathology
- Finding better means of undertaking cooperative studies with neurology, e.g., into the possible improvement of diagnosis
- Making more effective use of noninvasive imaging methods, since EEG studies are insufficient on their own
- Investigating more thoroughly the actions of carbamazepine – in epilepsy, affective disorder, trigeminal neuralgia
- Finding physiological or biochemical expressions of the genotype, at more fundamental levels than that of psychosis
- Finding ways of reducing the social disadvantage suffered by epileptic patients, particularly children and adolescents

The psychiatric effects of nonpsychiatric drugs were thought to require further research in five main directions: better methods of recording their unwanted effects, particularly in the elderly; development of simple measuring instruments; improving the sensitivity of doctors to identifying unwanted effects on cognition, mood, etc., including the encouragement of better drug histories; devising better experimental designs to determine whether symptoms caused by drugs can be separated from those caused by illness; and reexamining common drugs and the medication used in common conditions for possible psychiatric effects.

Finally, nine priorities were drawn up to constitute a European research agenda on the relationship of physical and psychiatric disorders:

- Implementation of existing knowledge, e.g., on rehabilitation of the brain-damaged
- Clinical and neurophysiological study of epilepsy, with emphasis on the use of new imaging methods
- In the case of AIDS, investigation of the neuropsychiatric aspects, of the implications of recent progress in immunology and virology, and of the effectiveness of educational methods related to the disorder
- More specific pharmacological studies, e.g., of cabamazepine and glutamates
- Improving awareness among health professionals of psychiatric problems resulting from the use of high-technology techniques in medicine
- Resolving the contradictory findings that have been obtained on causes of death in psychiatric patients
- Investigation of coping behaviors, including denial, which are found in serious physical disorders
- Improving the sensitivity of doctors to the psychiatric unwanted effects of nonpsychiatric drugs
- Further investigation of psychological influences on immunological processes

Subject Index

MIX
Papier aus verantwortungsvollen Quellen
Paper from responsible sources
FSC® C105338

If you have any concerns about our products,
you can contact us on
ProductSafety@springernature.com

In case Publisher is established outside the EU,
the EU authorized representative is:
Springer Nature Customer Service Center GmbH
Europaplatz 3, 69115 Heidelberg, Germany

Printed by Libri Plureos GmbH
in Hamburg, Germany